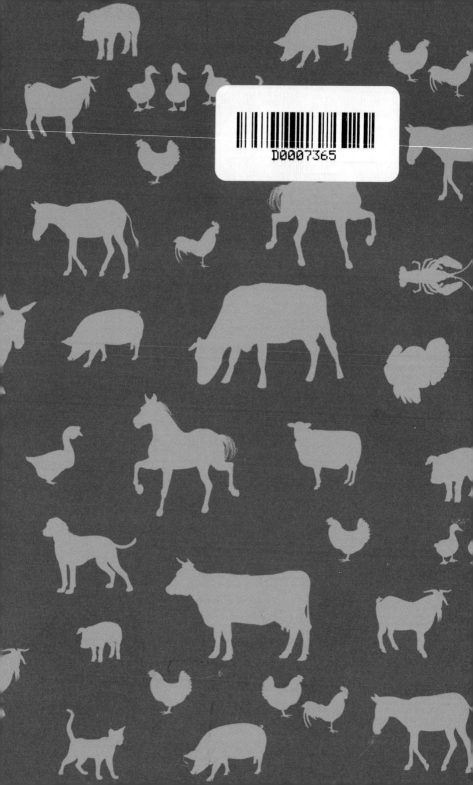

CREATURES OF THE ROCK

ANDREW PEACOCK

Creatures

OF THE

Rock

A VETERINARIAN'S

Adventures in

NEWFOUNDLAND

Doubleday Canada

Doubleday Canada and colophon are registered trademarks of Random House of Canada Limited

Library and Archives Canada Cataloguing in Publication

Peacock, Andrew (Veterinarian), author
Creatures of the rock : a veterinarian's adventures in Newfoundland / Andrew Peacock.

Includes bibliographical references and index.
Issued in print and electronic formats.
ISBN 978-0-385-68259-6

eBook ISBN 978-0-385-68260-2

1. Peacock, Andrew (Veterinarian). 2. Veterinarians—Newfoundland and Labrador—Biography. 3. Newfoundland and Labrador—Biography. I. Title.

SF613.P43A3 2014   636.089092   C2014-903159-9
                                                C2014-903160-2

Text images: (i) Darren Whittingham /Shutterstock.com; (iii, xi) © Andrey Churakov | Dreamstime.com; (284) © Tatiana Oleshkevich | Dreamstime.com. Endpaper images: © Andrey Churakov | Dreamstime.com and © Tatiana Oleshkevich | Dreamstime.com. Cover images: (boots) Simon Belcher/Getty Images; (chick) © Alptraum | Dreamstime.com; (stethoscope) © Janks | Dreamstime.com

Printed and bound in the USA

Published in Canada by Doubleday Canada, a division of Random House of Canada Limited, a Penguin Random House Company

www.randomhouse.ca

10 9 8 7 6 5 4 3 2

for Ingrid

"We can judge the heart of a man by his treatment of animals."

—IMMANUEL KANT

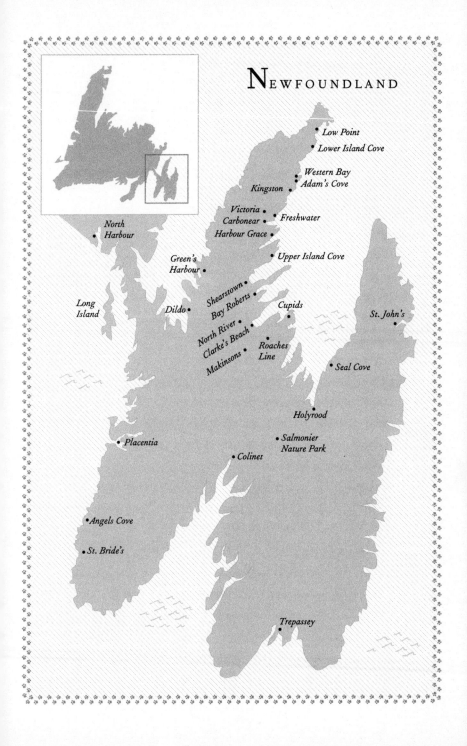

Newfoundland

Contents

Everything written in this book actually happened. Or if not, then something very much like it.

The stories range over much of my career but have a focus on the early years of settling in. Some of the accounts are conflations of real events. In some cases I have relocated a story: a calving may be accurately described but set in a different place in my practice. The names of most of my clients have been changed. My family; my secretary, Sharon; our two Australian shepherds, Pogo and Mats; and a few other characters in the book are very real people and dogs.

I love the language, idioms and accents of Newfoundland and have tried my best to capture them. This explains the occasional run-on sentence (not all Newfoundlanders speak slowly enough to allow for periods, or even sometimes commas). Inconsistencies in manner of speech reflect the variety of sub-dialects throughout my practice.

The content of the dialogue is of course somewhat approximate. It would be impossible to recreate word-for-word discussions from many years ago.

Beyond these details, it's all true.

Prologue

THE FREEZING RAIN SMASHED into the windshield in horizontal blasts. With every bend in the highway, the truck and I argued whether we should be on the road or in the ditch. Surely no lame horse was worth this treacherous trip.

The weather was bad enough that I had assumed there would be no calls that day. It would be a slow morning filled with paperwork in the office. One quick phone call put an end to that prospect. The language was English, I was pretty sure, but it took great concentration to discern that a horse belonging to a Mr. Green of Green's Harbour was "some terrible crippled, and right nish." I asked three times for directions, but my ear for the language of Newfoundland was not yet developed and I suspected Mr. Green had neglected to put in his teeth for our discussion. I would have to ask the way to Mr. Green's place when I got to Green's Harbour.

I had been in Newfoundland for less than two months, but I knew enough of the geography to find my way to most of the towns in my practice. Green's Harbour was on the other side of the peninsula where I lived and normally less than an hour away. Carefully creeping along the slick roads, I had little time to admire the sparkling ice jackets the freezing rain had left on the trees. This time it took nearly two hours to arrive in the village.

My first stop was at a small convenience store. The place was somehow simultaneously spotless and cluttered. The shelves were packed with every imaginable type of canned food. A homemade doll and an enormous round of bologna vied for space on the counter. Nowhere was there a speck of dirt. A short woman with white hair tied up in a loose bun sat knitting a sock behind the counter.

"Wonderful storm out there sir."

I loved the way Newfoundlanders used language. *Wonderful* didn't mean the same thing here as it did back in mainland Canada. Here the word was used more the way it was originally intended. Wonderful was something that filled you with wonder.

"Can you tell me where Mr. Green lives?"

"My son, we're all Green around here."

It took some time, but I eventually found out where Mr. Green with the crippled horse lived. It turned out that his name was Elihu and he lived next door to the shop. The woman behind the counter was his wife.

I left the truck where it was parked and carefully walked over the ice to the unpainted shed. Inside, the familiar warm heat from sheltered animals was a welcome relief from the freezing rain. There were three men and a horse in the barn. The horse was the only one without a cigarette going.

"You must be the vet."

"I am. Glad to meet you, Mr. Green."

"Good morning to you sir."

"This must be your horse with the bad leg."

"No sir."

The abruptness of this unexpected reply left me a little taken aback. "So . . . you have another horse somewhere that I should be looking at?"

"No sir."

"Sorry, I don't understand. You're Mr. Green, and this is your horse, right?"

"Ah we're havin' you on Doc. I'm Mr. Green but she's not my harse. I'm Calvin Green. This here's Elihu and she's his harse."

He pointed with his cigarette at a man back from the small crowd sitting on an overturned plastic salt-meat container. Everything made sense now and everyone had had a chance to have a little fun at my expense.

I went over to Elihu and asked him what the trouble was.

"Queen's been terrible crippled since sometime last week."

"Let's have a look at her."

Queen was a beautiful jet-black Newfoundland pony. I stepped into her stall and ran my hand along the side of her neck. Her skin was warm and comforting to the touch, and she turned calmly to watch me. After introducing myself by rubbing her eyelid and speaking quietly, I reached down and picked up her front left foot.

Right away I could see that her problem had been caused by overzealous trimming of her hooves. All such cutting should be done from the bottom. Cutting from the top or sides exposes sensitive parts to trauma and pain. Queen's hooves had been hacked at from the sides.

"Do you trim Queen's feet yourself, Elihu?"

"Yep."

"Can you tell me exactly how you do it?"

"Well, she's as quiet as an old dog, so she's not much trouble. I puts her foot up on a block of wood and cuts around the edge of her foot with an axe."

I tried to hide my cringe. "You know, Elihu, when you trim a horse's feet you should do it from the bottom. Here, let me show you with a hoof knife."

As I reached into my back pocket for a knife, Calvin Green pushed off from his resting spot against the barn wall and stepped directly in front of me.

"Skipper, this is the way we've all cut our horses' feet for fifty years. We've been doin' this since before you were born."

I hesitated in my reach for Queen's leg and thought for a minute. This was the first true challenge to my new position as vet. It was important for me to be on good terms with my clients, but it was more important that I helped them to look after their animals properly. I took a deep breath and looked from Calvin to Elihu.

"Guys, if you've been cutting feet like that for fifty years, you've been doing it wrong for fifty years. Now how would you like me to show you how you can trim Queen's feet without making her sore?"

It seemed as if the barn was silent for a minute or more.

Eventually Elihu pulled his hand out of his pocket and rubbed his cap around over his head. "Okay, Doc, let's see how you do it."

The trimming went well, and judging from the questions

asked, everyone in the barn had come around to being gen-uinely interested in the new method. Before I finished, I had Elihu make a couple of cuts around the bottom of the hoof. His smile betrayed his satisfaction with mastering the new technique.

After paying his bill, Elihu asked me if I liked salt fish. I told him I hadn't yet tried this Newfoundland delicacy. With a big, friendly smile, he handed me a thin triangular leathery-looking piece of material with a tail and fins. It smelled vaguely like old socks. As I started the truck and drove away from the farm, I wondered how I had ever ended up in such a strange and wonderful place.

For now, though, I had to figure out what to do with that fish.

1. The Pants of Destiny

MISS LENNOX WAS MY FAVOURITE teacher in elementary school. On first impression she didn't look the type to impress a young boy—she was a slow, bosomy woman with eyeglasses on a string and greying hair tied up in a severe bun. But Miss Lennox was relentlessly inquisitive. And she let us cut up frogs.

I remember distinctly the tangy mixture of excitement and disgust when we were first given our preserved frogs for dissection. The formaldehyde made our eyes sting as we set about cutting into an animal and poking around in its guts.

Whether it was from Miss Lennox's direction and example, or because I had a natural curiosity to match her own, I couldn't get enough of frog dissection. There inside the grey-green flesh was not a disgusting mess but a collection of organs and blood vessels. All of them had names and all of them did something complicated. I knew that what we learned in grade three science was only a peek into the marvels of what made an animal tick.

Even before I encountered Miss Lennox, I had enjoyed the company of animals. My summers were spent on my grandfather's farm where the dog was a constant companion and the cattle were everyone's concern. From a young age I was fascinated by the creatures that existed alongside us but that lived a different life and saw the world in a different way.

Students often say they want to be veterinarians because they love animals. Any vet will tell you this isn't enough. In order to be a good vet and to enjoy that kind of work, I believe a person first needs an unquenchable curiosity about animals. Good vets want to know about the things that make an animal work and how to fix whatever interferes with those workings. I think the very best vets also want to know about how animals think, and realize it isn't much like the way we think.

At about thirteen years old, I got my first real taste of veterinary medicine. Before that time, I wasn't allowed out in the barn when the vet came to my grandfather's farm. General consensus was that I would be in the way and I wouldn't be interested in what went on out there anyway. It didn't cool my curiosity to see my dad and grandfather return from the barn splattered with blood after dehornings.

One crisp fall day, the local vet, Doc Davey, came to see whether my grandfather's cows were pregnant. There was to be no blood or dangerous procedures, so I was allowed to come out to the barn and watch. Doc Davey wasn't a big man, but his friendly manner, knowledge and skill made him huge in my eyes. He talked politics for a while and laughed in a way that made it apparent that he thought that anyone who was involved in that business or followed it too closely was a little simple.

My father led the first cow into a stall and fastened its head. The vet pulled on a plastic glove that nearly went to his shoulder and squirted lubricant on his hand. Next, he held the tail in his ungloved hand and stuck his covered arm right up the cow's back end! I could hardly believe my eyes. The same mixture of revulsion and curiosity that I had experienced in grade three washed over me. Why would anyone want to do such a thing? And more importantly, what was he looking for in there? The vet explained that he was feeling the cow's uterus and could tell from its texture whether a calf was developing.

I was hooked. It was one thing to mess around in the guts of a dead frog, but here was a man reaching inside a live animal, feeling around and coming back with useful information. To me it was a true hero's journey. From that moment on, I knew that this was what I wanted to do.

Veterinary medicine let you scratch that itch of curiosity about animals, and do so in pleasant surroundings. This was no job behind a desk or stuck in a building in a city. As well as the intellectual stimulation, there was fresh air to breathe, real physical work to do and fascinating people to work with and help. Where else could anyone find such a satisfying mix?

University was another experience. Moving away from home and learning to balance new-found freedoms with the need to study were hard. Many of the courses I took were interesting, but in the back of my mind I wished I could skip all that and get right down to going to farms and fixing animals.

After four years of studying basic science, I applied to veterinary school. When told I had an interview, I understood I was facing one of the most important moments in my life. Lots of people wanted to be vets. There had to be dozens if not hundreds of candidates for every position available. In the space of less than an hour I would have to convince my interviewers that I should be one of the favoured ones.

To prepare, I read everything that I could find about veterinary medicine. I learned a bit about everything, from the history of the profession to what were the main mastitis-causing bacteria. It was soon obvious that no amount of study was going to impress anyone with my knowledge of veterinary medicine. More importantly, I had to demonstrate somehow that my personality would fit this world.

What better way is there to show who you are, I reasoned, than with clothes? Normally I don't pay much attention to fashion. Clothes are to keep you warm and dry, and if they are easy to clean, that's enough. For this one shining day, though, I decided that my attire would take on a special role and accurately say who I was.

These clothes would have to state in no uncertain terms how seriously I took this interview. This was no whim; it was a potential turning point in my life. Perhaps a suit would give this impression. But then again, a suit might not suggest the wearer was someone willing to roll up his sleeves and do the dirty work that farm animal practice often involved.

I concluded that a good compromise would be to wear a white shirt and tie with a sweater and neatly pressed wool pants. The more I considered the details of my apparel, the more important they became in the whole story of my interview. Eventually I decided that I needed a simple red tie, a sky-blue sweater and navy blue pants.

I already had the blue sweater. It was easy to find a red tie and a crisp new white shirt. The pants were another story.

By the weekend before the interview, I hadn't found any pants that met my rather strict self-imposed dress code. The interview was on Monday, and Saturday was my last chance to find the finishing touches for an outfit that I was coming to think would be critical to my success.

I was fortunate to have my girlfriend, Ingrid, visiting me this important weekend. We had met two years earlier, at a training course for a summer job, and she was presently in medical school in Ottawa, three hundred miles away. We shared a fascination with medicine, music and the outdoors and a lack of interest in fashion. Still, I felt that having a woman along might help avoid a serious wardrobe blunder. Starting on Saturday morning, the two of us combed through every men's clothing store in Guelph.

As closing time approached, and with one last store to visit, the chances for success were looking bleak. If we didn't find the pants now, my plans for sartorial splendour were surely down the drain—along with all hope of becoming a veterinarian.

As I walked to the rack of trousers in that final store, my heart was falling. What were the chances that this establishment stocked what no other place in the city of Guelph had to offer? Leafing through the navy blue pants, I couldn't see anything appropriate.

A sales assistant approached us.

I described the size, material and colour I was looking for, and he ruffled through the same pants I had just looked through.

"Sorry, nothing like that here. I'd suggest you try the place down the street but they'll be closed by the time you get there."

Failure had landed with a sickening dull thud.

The man must have seen the dejected look on my face. "Are these the kind of pants you're looking for?" he asked, holding open his sports jacket and looking down at his own.

"Yes. That's exactly what I wanted." The fact that I could now see the unattainable pants was not helping.

"Would you like these?"

My head snapped up. "What?"

"I bought them yesterday, and if you like, I'll get them cleaned and you can pick them up next week."

"That's amazing, but I need them for Monday morning."

"No problem. Give me your address. I'll get them cleaned tonight and bring them around to your place tomorrow."

I didn't hug him, but I was tempted. I paid for the pants, and we walked home in triumph.

On Monday morning, I had my new pants and I was ready for the interview. Sitting with all the other suited candidates in a waiting room, I reflected on how they didn't look like they would be much good with a cow. Even the thin-haired girl running from the interview room crying couldn't dampen my optimistic enthusiasm. She'd been wearing a serious-looking business ensemble too.

The interview itself was a bit of a blur. The three veterinarians were friendly and asked reasonable questions of a general nature. They asked only one technical question. Unbelievably, they asked what bacteria are the most common cause of mastitis. As the interview drew down to its conclusion, I was feeling optimistic. I had been given a fair chance to show who I was and I had done it to the best of my ability. If they liked me, I would be in vet school.

Just before we were finished, one of the vets leaned forward, drummed ten digits across the table once from pinkies to thumbs, and asked a final question.

"How did you decide what you were going to wear today?"

I told them my reasons for my outfit and then the story of my quest for the pants. They all laughed and told me it had been a pleasure talking to me.

I'm convinced that when the assessors went through their interview summaries to decide who would get into vet school, someone stopped when they got to my page.

"That was the guy with the pants, wasn't it? He was all right, wasn't he?"

That's all it would take, some way to stand out. In the end, I was right about the interview. The clothes were important, and getting exactly the right pants had been critical.

2. A Complete Boar

THE FIRST CHANCE THAT students get to act like a real veterinarian is during their last summer vacation before graduating. Most will apply for work experience, which can vary anywhere from cleaning out kennels to full-blown practice. My classmate Greg and I were lucky enough to find work with a practice in Kapuskasing, in northern Ontario. As well as serving the pet-owning population of this town of twelve thousand, the veterinary practice looked after all of the farm animals for nearly a hundred miles in every direction. All this work was done by one veterinarian. To say the least, he was overstretched and welcomed the relief that competent students could offer in the summer.

Dr. Bob Wright, a slim man of impeccable manner and dress, had been alone in the practice for over ten years. In his solitude, he had developed his own way of practice. As long as students showed they weren't complete incompetents and subscribed to his ideas of how things should be done, he was great to work for. From the first days on the job, Greg and I were allowed to help in surgery. As Bob's confidence in us developed, we were encouraged to do more and more on our own. Within a month of starting, the two of us were going out on minor farm calls without supervision.

Late one Friday afternoon, Bob had left and Greg and I were cleaning up the clinic. We had the keenness of those given new respect and took every chance to hang around the office. I answered a phone call from the town of Moonbeam asking if we could castrate the caller's pig. This type of routine call would normally be relegated to weekday work, but in my exuberance I immediately agreed to see to it on Saturday morning.

"Tomorrow?"

"Sure, we can come out first thing."

"You are coming to castrate my pig"—there was a pause—"tomorrow morning?"

I was a little taken aback. "You sound surprised."

"Well, yeah. The doc's been putting this job off for nearly three years now."

I paused to consider the implications. This pig had to be at least three years old. My assumption had been that this was a routine castration of a newborn pig, a simple procedure fit to be done by a couple of green students. Piglets are easy to handle and don't require anaesthesia. An adult boar is an altogether different story.

"Uh, how heavy do you think your pig is, sir?"

"I'd say she's at least six hundred pounds."

"She" was a very big boar, and this was not going to be a simple procedure. Still, I had committed us and I wasn't about to back away from a challenge so early in my career. I got directions to the farm and hung up.

"Hey, Greg, you got any idea how you would castrate a six-hundred-pound boar?"

"Nope, don't remember anything about that."

"Well, we're doing one tomorrow morning."

The two of us spent most of the night looking through our ever-present school notes. The only reference we could find was that pigs could be anaesthetized for minor surgeries by injecting barbiturates into their ear veins. This procedure was recommended for animals up to 175 pounds. We were short about four hundred pounds.

With the knowledge from our notes exhausted, we turned to the clinic's library. We started poring over Bob's back issues of various journals, and after nearly an hour, Greg called out that he had something: an anecdotal reference to a veterinarian castrating a large boar by injecting one of its testicles with a solution formulated for euthanizing dogs. Once injected, went the theory, the solution would be slowly drawn up into the general circulation by the blood vessels supplying the area. When the animal lost consciousness, the testicles were to be quickly removed to make sure the dose was cut off too, before it became lethal.

Our youthful enthusiasm made this seem like a good idea.

We arrived at the Moonbeam farm first thing Saturday morning ready to put our questionable anaesthetic technique to use. A number of neighbours had gathered to watch. The farmer, Jacques, obviously wanted to share his joy that someone had at last come to straighten out his pig.

This was disconcerting. Maybe we were up to the job, but there was no way we were ready to perform for an audience.

We exchanged pleasantries and asked where our patient was.

"She's up in that shed." Jacques pointed to a small raised building close to where we had parked.

"Okay, let's have a look."

I am sure that Greg, like me, felt the combined power and responsibility of our newly assumed status as we pulled on our coveralls. These people had come to watch professionals at work and we had better not disappoint.

The shed was not much bigger than ten feet square and raised nearly three feet off the ground. Strange accommodation for an adult boar, I thought. We opened the door tentatively—then slammed it shut when the monster inside charged toward us. Greg and I regrouped away from the crowd and admitted to each other that we had no idea how to restrain this animal long enough to administer the anaesthetic. Perhaps Jacques could be of some assistance.

"Hey, Jacques. Do you ever bring that boar outside?"

"Are you kidding? She would kill us if you let her loose."

So Jacques wouldn't be much help. We snuck back up to the shed and shifted an old oil drum over so we could climb up and look in through the window. The boar's housing was worse than we thought. Not only was the space small, but there were a few floorboards missing near the middle, over a manure pit below. This may have been designed for waste removal, but it looked suspiciously like a trap for vet students. Entering the boar's lair would one way or another be suicidal.

Greg suggested luring out the boar with feed and capturing him with ropes cleverly positioned nearby. We reasoned that once he started into eating, we could pull the ropes up around his body for a harness of some type. Both of us agreed that this was a good idea.

Jacques brought us a pail of pig feed and we placed a small pile just in front of the pig's residence. Next we laid a twenty-foot length of rope along the ground between this bait and the front door. It never crossed our minds that failure could result in a near-feral boar rampaging on the loose.

Somehow, the boar co-operated. When we opened the shed door he jumped out and ignored us as he made a bee-line for the feed. Luck was with us as he stopped perfectly positioned over our rope. We made a small loop in one end and passed the other tip through. With a slight tug we had a noose around the boar's chest. He was preoccupied enough with the feed to allow us one more loop in front of his front legs. We had a perfectly adequate harness around the boar and absolutely no idea what to do next.

The pig slobbered through the pile of feed and started to run. Greg and I grabbed the end of the rope and soon discovered that two slight vet students could not hold a hurtling six-hundred-pound boar. We dug in our heels and slid a few feet before deciding, much to the delight of the assembled onlookers, that running with the pig was the only chance to stay with the rope.

It was hard to blame the animal for wanting to run. His shed was woefully inadequate and the freedom of the open yard must have been intoxicating. Unfortunately, he started off in the direction of the highway in front of Jacques's house. As we came up to a telephone pole, it occurred to me that this could provide an anchor to the runaway pig. With the rope secured by two quick throws around the pole, the boar came to a screeching halt.

The animal was now in a swampy area just off the road. It didn't seem an appropriate venue for a castration. Our next challenge was to move him to the relatively clean gravel drive and find a place to secure him. As there were no posts or other solid vertical structures in the area, we decided that the bumper of our van would do.

To make sure we didn't lose the boar in the relocation, we used another long rope to tie its harness to the bumper. Now we had to persuade the creature to move.

In vet school our studies included training in the necessary art of handling animals. I remember being told that if you knew what you were doing, a horse would go the way you wanted one hundred percent of the time. With a cow, this decreased to fifty percent. But a pig would always go in the opposite direction.

The only way to overcome this natural obstinacy is to be smarter than the pig. The standard method is to put a bucket of feed over its face and back the pig up. Convince a pig you would like it to move forward and it will happily oblige by shifting into reverse. Jacques provided another bucket of snacks, and with some crafty steering we had the boar fastened on close to the van.

The pig was so thrilled with the feed that he didn't notice us washing up his back end in preparation for the surgery. As previously agreed, Greg would administer the anaesthetic and I would do the cutting.

My partner retrieved the dog-euthanizing drug from the

van and filled a syringe with the appropriate amount. I held the bucket over the pig's face while Greg moved around behind the animal.

Injecting a drug into a testicle should be a simple procedure, especially on an animal as well endowed as this boar. There were no veins to find or nerves to avoid. But then Greg jumped up shaking his arm and swearing.

"What happened?"

"The bugger moved and I stuck the needle into my thumb."

From time to time in the heat of the moment, a vet will stick a needle into himself. When this happens, it is best if the drug involved is not a poison. Greg continued to hop up and down sucking on his thumb.

"You gonna be okay?"

"Yeah, yeah. It just stung a bit."

Greg bent over again and this time injected the pig's testicle.

The article we'd read didn't go into great detail about how the anaesthetic worked. We found out why. Shortly after the injection, the pig started to shake. The shaking progressed to the point where it would be best described as a conniption fit if not a convulsion. The van rocked from side to side until I seriously worried that the vehicle might topple.

As the pig's writhing subsided, his legs gave way and he tumbled onto his back. I stepped over his abdomen so that I was standing with one leg on either side of him, facing his tail. I took an iodine-soaked swab, did a final prep on the surgical site and picked up a scalpel. Bending over the supine pig's belly, I made a deep cut along the length of the scrotum. A single testicle popped out ready for removal.

I reached an arm out. "Hey, Greg, hand me the emasculators."

There was no answer. I straightened up and looked for my partner. Greg wasn't standing behind the pig and I didn't see him among the onlookers. Immediately, I worried that he was lying in the grass somewhere, victim of the self-injection of a dog-killing drug. Greg's health was a problem, but in my zeal for professionalism I decided that the job at hand required my first attention. The testicles needed prompt removal before toxic levels of drug built up and killed our patient.

I called out to a teenager leaning against our van.

"Hey, can you hand me that thing that looks like a big pair of pliers?"

"What?"

Time was ticking by for the pig and perhaps for Greg. "Quick, those things right there." I pointed to the emasculators just beyond my reach.

"Okay, man, just relax."

Perhaps my voice betrayed the sense of urgency or even panic that I felt. Still, the teenage boy was not to be hurried. In a frustrating display of slow motion, he drew himself up from his slouch against the van and ambled the five feet to the instrument.

When I finally got the instrument, I made short work of cutting and crushing the vessels and tissue that connected the testicle to the pig. In no time, I had the second testicle exposed and removed. Now it was time to find my partner.

As I stepped across the pig I saw Greg coming around the corner of Jacques's house. In his hand was a roll of paper towels.

"I thought you might want some of these."

If I wasn't so happy to see my friend alive, I could have killed him. As it would be unprofessional to show my true feelings, I took a piece of paper towel and dabbed unnecessarily at the surgical wound.

The procedure hadn't exactly gone as we had planned, but we had accomplished our first complicated job. All that remained was for the pig to wake up.

We wrote a bill and chatted and the pig snored. We went inside for a cup of coffee and still the animal slept. After nearly an hour, we decided we were not much help watching the slumbering pig. As the temperature was rising, we gave instructions for Jacques to put some temporary shade over the boar to keep the sun off and to occasionally spray him with water.

Apart from a thumb that went numb for several hours, Greg had no ill effects from our adventure. We found out that night that it took over six hours for the pig to wake up. Intra-testicular injection of dog-euthanasia solution had proved workable for large boar castration. The procedure was successful and I would never attempt it again.

3. Coming to the Rock

AFTER WE'D FOUND THE perfect pants together, my relationship with Ingrid grew. Two years into vet school we were married on a hill overlooking a southern Ontario beef farm. We had fabulous adventures during the summers, but most of the year we were still in schools separated by hundreds of miles. Both of us were anxious to be done with school and begin our lives together in one place.

Finally, I finished my time at the Ontario Veterinary College in Guelph. I had learned the basic science required to understand veterinary medicine and a few of the practical skills needed to head out into the world of animal repair.

These four years culminated in a sadistic ritual known as the orals. Students who'd survived this far were taken into a small room where two professors asked questions about what they had been taught and in some cases about things they had not been taught. Tales of impossibly difficult grillings and the resulting nervous breakdowns were part of the shared mythology of the school from the moment new students arrived.

The one positive aspect of the orals was that they signalled the end of school. Once they were over, it was time to get out into the real world and do what most of us had wanted to be doing for a very long time. It was also around oral time that many students found the jobs that would start their adventures in veterinary medicine.

It had never occurred to me that being married to a medical doctor would be an obstacle in my search for employment.

At first I considered returning to my home town of Kapuskasing in northern Ontario. The previous summer I had worked there with Dr. Wright, and he was now looking for an associate. Ingrid looked for employment in the town, but found that Kapuskasing had no need for a new doctor.

I then considered northern Saskatchewan. I spoke with a vet in a remote area who was interested in having me come up to work with her. The practice sounded exciting, a mix of small and large animals in a wilderness setting. Again, we ran into problems with Ingrid finding work. The practice was based in a town with one older doctor who had been the only show in town for decades. Ingrid contacted him, but he made it clear that he would do everything in his power to make life difficult for any new young female who intruded on his territory. Neither of us was interested in starting our careers in that kind of atmosphere.

Standing in a cold hall waiting for my oral exam on small animals, I spotted a notice pinned to a bulletin board. The Government of Newfoundland was looking for a vet to work in a farm animal practice. I liked the idea of kicking off my career with an exciting adventure, and took down the phone number.

Later that night, I spoke with a sophisticated-sounding man who was the provincial veterinarian. An interview was arranged for the following week, when a delegation from Newfoundland would be coming to the college to find a vet.

I knew almost nothing about Newfoundland. I understood that it was an island off the east coast of Canada where people spoke in an odd way and life was a little less sophisticated than in the rest of the country. Every year at the student awards at the college, there were patronizing titters when it came time to give out the Conception Bay Kennel Club award for top student from Newfoundland in third year. There was never much suspense around who would win, as there never seemed to be more than one student from Newfoundland in third year.

The job interview went well. The men I spoke with were pleasant and painted an appealing picture of the position in rural Newfoundland. My strongest impression from the meeting came when one of the interviewers took out a map and swept his hand across it to show the extent of the practice under discussion. It was indeed immense, but what really caught my eye was the name of the town his index finger came to rest on: Dildo.

That night, I got a phone call saying that the job was mine if I was interested. When I said I was available as long as Ingrid could find work, I was told that the government would fly us to the province to see the practice and look into employment for my wife.

Two weeks later we arrived in Newfoundland. We were taken to the main agricultural office in St. John's for a quick tour and then driven to the town of Harbour Grace, where the practice was based. The journey had its own stark beauty. Long stretches of boulders and moss stretched out from the highway to a distant foggy ocean coast. The tundra-like bleakness reminded me of the landscape I had encountered when I worked as a student in Inuit villages in far northern Quebec.

We were first taken to a modern-looking hotel in Harbour Grace that didn't take credit cards. Next we went to the office I would be working out of and were left in the care of the staff. Ingrid spoke with the doctors in the office upstairs, and plans were made to have her join their practice. Everyone in the agriculture office was friendly beyond anything that I had seen in mainland Canada. The secretary, Sharon, had a sparkle in her eyes and more than gave back the teasing she got from the men in the office. After an afternoon talking with the staff, we were invited by the local agricultural representative, Blake, for a meal at his house in Adam's Cove.

We climbed into his truck and drove to the wharf around the corner from the office. He spoke with two men who were cleaning fish and soon had an enormous cod to take home for supper.

The half-hour drive to Blake's house only reinforced our infatuation with the place. The road twisted through small villages dotted with houses covered in brightly painted clapboard. There were few trees, but many dramatic rock outcroppings and amazing views of the ocean.

The only concern I had was the apparent lack of animals. When I asked Blake about this, he was reassuring.

"There are lots of them around here. That's Johnny Weston's place. See the barn out behind the house? He keeps four cows and a half-dozen goats in there over the winter. They're all out on pasture for the summer. You have to get off the road to see the livestock. See that place there? That's Will John Johnson's. He has sheep, but you won't likely hear much from him. He keeps to himself."

We arrived at Blake's place to find a refurbished traditional old house right on the ocean. The views from the house were spectacular. Blake and his wife had done the renovations themselves. Everything inside, including the kitchen cupboards, had a homemade earthy feel. It wasn't the finest carpentry in the world, yet the whole house exuded a warmth that won us over. After a home-cooked meal and much pleasant conversation, Ingrid and I both felt we had seen a model for our future in that house.

The next morning we were driven back to St. John's. I told the provincial vet that everything was fine and we were ready to move and start work. We were told that all of our moving expenses would be paid, so long as we stayed for two years.

Ingrid and I had our first jobs. We agreed we would work in rural Newfoundland for two years and then move on to further adventures.

4. First Call

INGRID AND I EACH DROVE a car from Ontario to Newfoundland and started looking for a house to rent in the town of Carbonear. Our first surprise was how cheap the rents were around the bay. We found a delightful six-bedroom house for under three hundred dollars a month. The stately nature of the old yellow clapboard house and the lazy, tree-lined road it was on were of more interest to us than the fact that a young couple didn't really need six bedrooms. All that was missing was an ocean view.

After settling in and reacquainting myself with the people I would be working with, I was driven into the city of St. John's to pick up my vet truck. Fresh out of school, I think I was expecting some kind of imparting of wisdom before I started work. Vet school had filled my head with skills and facts, but I wasn't sure that I had a clue how actually to be a veterinarian. I was also the only graduate from my class to be going into practice solo. Everyone else had had the sense to kick off their careers under the direction of someone more experienced. My practice was a two-hour drive from the nearest veteran vet.

My orientation was short and direct. As I walked into my boss's office, he rose from behind his desk, straightened his jacket and shook my hand.

"I'm delighted that you've chosen to come and work with us. Here's a map of your practice." He twisted around and pointed out the window behind his desk. "That yellow Jimmy is yours. Here are the keys. Drop in again sometime. Oh, and before you go, you'd better check with the secretary to see if you have any calls to do today." At the secretary's desk, I found that there was indeed work waiting for me. She had spoken with Owen Prince in Cupids and let him know that I would be along that day to see his cut horse. The secretary had helpfully written out directions to find the animal, so I was ready to go. I didn't tell the secretary that I had no idea where the town of Cupids was. Instead, I sat in my truck and unfolded the map of the province. It didn't take long to find the town; it was directly on my way home from St. John's. As I pulled out of the office lot, I wondered what kind of cut this would be and how I would manage to close it up. I worried that I'd never actually knocked a horse out with drugs.

The road from St. John's to Cupids was a meandering route that skirted along the edge of Conception Bay. The scenery amazed, the sun dazzled and colourful saltbox houses lined the ocean's edge. I had a sudden impression I was being paid to be a tourist. This was nothing like the straight flat roads lined with conifers that I had left behind in northern Ontario. Dramatic outcroppings of rock and spectacular ocean views passed by until I came to a sign announcing Cupids.

Enough of this sightseeing—it was time to be a vet. My instructions told me to head down the main road into Cupids and turn right at the bottom of the harbour; the horse was right next to the water. It sounded simple enough. I followed the main road in until I reached the ocean. There was no right turn so I continued straight. The first right turn was nearly a quarter mile beyond what I would have called the bottom of the harbour, and there was no horse in sight anywhere near.

I pulled up beside a woman walking along the road and rolled down my window. "Hi. Can you tell me where Mr. Prince lives? He has a horse I'm supposed to see."

"My son, you're way off your port."

The accent was thick and the terms were foreign to me, but I understood I was nowhere near where I should be.

"Could you tell me where Mr. Prince is?"

"Yes my darlin'. You just head right back where you came from and turn right when you gets to the end of the water. The 'arse is right there."

My mistake was obvious. The turn *was* to the right, but it was a right turn to be taken *after* driving by the place and coming back again. I turned the truck around and headed back for the bottom of the harbour.

When I made the proper turn, there was indeed a short brown horse with a black mane and tail standing out near the water. I pulled up the truck and walked up to the house nearest the animal. A stocky middle-aged woman with an infectious smile came out before I could knock.

"I thought that might be you drivin' by. Strange truck around here, ya know. We thought it odd that ya drove right by the house. That's Queen over there." She pointed to the horse.

We walked over and I rubbed Queen's face. She leaned into the pressure of my hand, enjoying the attention.

"So what's your trouble, sweetheart?"

"She's got a cut, right there on her shawolder."

I stepped around to the side Mrs. Prince had indicated and saw a cut about an inch long that didn't completely penetrate the skin. No one had ever said anything in vet school about treating a little cut like this. If this was a foot long and down into a couple of layers of muscle, I would know exactly how to deal with it. If this horse had some disease with a five- or six-syllable name, I would be ready to rhyme off regimens of drugs and management.

This little cut, this scratch, was something else. There was nothing here that I could suture and it wasn't deep enough that it would get infected. But this was my first call, and for my own self-esteem I had to act decisively.

"That's a nasty cut, Mrs. Prince. We better get that cleaned up. Can you get me a little warm water and some paper towel?"

As Mrs. Prince ambled back to her house, I went to the truck. I wondered whether Queen should get a shot of antibiotics. My education was going to be no help in dealing with this case; instead I quickly learned the one important fact that school had never emphasized. A lot of this work was going to be about simple common sense.

I thought for a minute. What would *I* do if I'd been cut like this? I wouldn't go to the doctor, it wouldn't get stitched and I wouldn't take an antibiotic. There certainly would be no way that I would get an injectable antibiotic. The only problem was that Mrs. Prince had called the vet and expected something concrete and maybe even a little spectacular to be done for her horse. She would be disappointed if I only cleaned up the cut.

Horses with cuts are very susceptible to tetanus, a terrible disease caused by bacteria commonly found in soil. It usually kills, after a prolonged period of pain and misery. Vaccination drastically diminishes a horse's chance of becoming infected. Queen was going to get a shot.

When Mrs. Prince and I met again next to Queen, I carefully cleaned around the cut with the water and paper towel supplied. Next, I soaked a cotton swab in iodine and rubbed it across the wound. With a slap, I placed a needle into the muscles of Queen's neck and delivered the tetanus vaccine.

"There you go, Mrs. Prince—Queen's all cleaned up and she has a shot to keep her from getting lockjaw."

"Thank you, Doctor. What would we do without a vet to help us when we gets in trouble like this? Owen told me it was a waste of time callin' you, but I knowed you could help Queen."

I wrote up a bill and got back into my truck. I had a happy client and I'd learned more in that one call than from a day spent poring over textbooks. I was going to be fine.

5. Gut Reaction

INGRID OFTEN CAME ALONG with me on calls on weekends and her days off. Our unusual hours, with my vet calls coming at any time of the day or night and her emergency shifts at the hospital, meant that we saw each other less than we would like.

One Saturday, I was called to see a "blown-up" cow on the other side of Conception Bay, in a community called Seal Cove. Ingrid was free for the day, so we decided to make a trip of it.

We took the old road around Conception Bay that sticks close to the ocean and winds up and down over the hills and through many villages. It was a warm and bright summer day, and as I admired the seacoast scenery, I kept thinking how great it was to have a job where I could go out on such a drive with my best friend.

The cow owner's house was easy to pick out, with its dark green clapboard and bright red trim. No one was in the yard and there was no answer when we knocked on the door. We wandered out behind the house and found a cow tied to a fence.

This had to be our patient. The cow looked as if someone had inflated her with a bicycle pump and that she might float away if she hadn't been fastened to the fence. As we walked around the poor grunting animal, we heard whistling and saw two men heading up the lane toward the house.

"You guys know who owns this cow?"

"She's mine, skipper," offered the shorter plump man with the baseball cap pulled tightly down to his ears. So this was Mike who had called in such a panic three-quarters of an hour ago.

"I'm the vet. You called me to come and see your cow."

The younger, thin man had a couple of teeth on prominent display over one side of his bottom lip. He started to laugh and then began a coughing fit that ended with him holding himself up by a fence post. With these preliminaries out of the way, he went into an episode of hacking and spitting that seemed to cure his cough.

"How long has she been looking like this?"

"I first noticed her lookin' a bit big yesterday morning," Mike told me, "and by yesterday afternoon the one side of her was blown way out. Now this morning she's out on both sides."

It was too bad the owner hadn't called me the previous day. The cow was suffering from bloat, and stuffed so tight with gas that she might now be damaged internally by the pressure. Untreated bloat can quickly prove fatal.

One big advantage that cows have over people is that they can eat grass, one of the most plentiful and easily grown plants on earth. It is difficult, however, to digest. Much of the bulk of grass is made up of cellulose, which takes so long to digest that cows have four stomachs for the purpose, known as the reticulum, rumen, omasum and abomasum. The largest stomach, the rumen, is filled with micro-organisms for breaking down cellulose, a process that creates a by-product of about twenty gallons of gas per cow per day.

As a result, cows are constantly belching. Some environmentalists think this belching is a major threat to the ozone layer. Not being able to burp, certainly, is a major threat to any cow. If the gas produced in cellulose digestion isn't passed, the rumen continues to fill up and the cow visibly enlarges.

Veterinarians divide the resulting bloats into the categories of "frothy" and "obstructive." The first comes about when bubbly indigestion prevents the cow from belching, much like what happens when soap bubbles refuse to go down the drain when a sink is emptied.

Obstructive bloat is simpler. When a cow belches, gas passes from the rumen through the esophagus and out the mouth. If anything solid gets stuck in the esophagus, gases become trapped.

The bloat in this cow was so advanced that I dispensed with the careful examination that's usual before any treatment. My first priority was to get the gas out and relieve this animal's obvious discomfort.

"We'll stick a tube down her throat first and see if we can deflate her."

As I hurried over to my truck, I noticed Mike's friend falling in a little too closely behind me. I wasn't comfortable with the way he avoided eye contact every time I looked his way. All of my clients I had encountered to this point had been a pleasure to work with, but this man gave me concern. I opened the back door of the fibreglass unit that carried my drugs and equipment, hauled out my boots and pulled them on. As I leaned down to tighten my footwear, I noticed him pulling open one of the unit's drawers.

"I could use some of these," he said as he grabbed a couple of syringes and a handful of needles and slipped them into the breast pocket of his well-worn and elbowless sports coat. He turned quickly and hurried toward the house.

I wasn't sure what he wanted the needles and syringes for, but I doubted that his interest was in treating animals. "Hey, buddy," I called. "Come here for a second."

He spun around and gave me a look somewhere in the murky ground between confusion and defiance. "What for?"

"Come here. I want to talk to you for a minute."

A little too fast for my liking, he strode back and planted himself with his face two feet from mine. "Okay, whaddaya want?"

"I'll tell you what," I said as I clapped him on the shoulder with a somewhat less than friendly hand. "These"—my hand moved down to his breast pocket and removed the syringes and needles—"stay here. I need them for the cows and horses."

I replaced his plunderings in my truck and braced myself for his response.

"Man, you are some cheap." He stalked away.

My actions hadn't won me a friend, but the idea of having someone take things from my truck while I stood by didn't sit well with me. I also didn't like the idea of becoming a supplier of needles and syringes to the local community.

With that out of the way, I pulled a speculum and a ten-foot flexible rubber hose called a stomach tube from the truck, locked up the back and returned to the cow.

The speculum is a two-foot-long piece of stainless steel tubing that looks like it would be at home on a vacuum cleaner. Its purpose is to keep cows from chewing on the stomach tube while it is down their throat. Chewing quickly ruins these tubes, and a tube with the end bitten off could be very difficult to retrieve from the esophagus and stomach.

I held the tube up against the side of the cow and measured the distance from her mouth to the back of her ribs. By marking this distance on the rubber with a piece of tape, I would know when the end had reached the rumen.

Quite understandably, cows resent metal tubes being put into their mouths and rubber tubes down their throats. Holding the cow's head, speculum and stomach tube in place often resulted in an interesting ride.

This animal was exhausted from the effects of the bloat and offered little resistance as I sidled up and wrapped my right arm around her head. With the fingers of my right hand, I was able to grab hold of the cow's tongue and pull it out the right side of her jaws. This caused her to open up her mouth, and with my free hand I placed the speculum in and pushed it to the back of her throat. Once the speculum is in place, cows always begin to chew. The metal tube is irritating, and they do everything they can with chewing motions and pushing with their tongue to remove this foreign body. All this mouth action causes the cow to profusely salivate until the procedure is finished. The resulting slime makes it even more difficult to keep a firm grip on the speculum.

Once the speculum was firmly in place, Ingrid handed me

the end of the stomach tube, which she had lubricated with a little mineral oil. The tube slid easily through the speculum and down the esophagus until the appearance of the tape indicated we were in far enough. Almost immediately a blast of foul-smelling gas erupted from the end of the tube.

I had a flashback to my days as a student travelling around with Dr. Wright in northern Ontario. One day while relieving a bloat by stomach tube, the vet had introduced me to the mysteries of lighting bloats. Because much of the gas in a cow's stomach is methane, it's very flammable. If a flame is held to the end of a tube releasing rumen gas, he explained, a spectacular blue flame ensues. He said that he had never tried it, but had heard of a veterinarian in Holland demonstrating this trick, only to burn down his client's barn and house. I could understand how this story kept him from lighting bloats inside his farmers' barns.

But this time, I had a bloated cow outside, with nothing flammable within a flame-thrower's reach. I couldn't let this opportunity pass.

"Have you got a lighter?" I asked Mike. "I can show you something really neat."

He patted his pockets and shook his head. "No, not on me. Wait now, I'll sing out for Darryl. *Darryl!* Get over here."

Mike's friend was now sitting on a stump with a bottle of beer in his hands. He pulled himself up, stretched and ambled over to the cow.

"Darryl, ya got a lighter?"

"Yeah, but I got no smokes on me."

"Forget the smokes. Give me your lighter."

Darryl passed over his lighter, and as he briefly looked in my direction, contempt flashed from his face.

"If you flick your lighter in front of this tube," I explained, "we'll get to see a beautiful blue flame."

"I'd like to see that," said Mike as he moved around to the front of the cow and ignited the lighter into the gas issuing from the tube.

The resulting whoosh told me that the gases had ignited, but the visual display was less than impressive. Instead of a blue flame, all I could see was an unusual shimmering around the end of the tube. Whatever gases were in this cow were burning colourlessly, and my display was a dismal letdown.

Darryl shifted closer to the tube. "I don't see no flame."

With this, he placed his face directly in front of the tube. He let out a little yelp and jerked his face back out of the heat. Without further comment, he walked back to his stump and returned his attentions to his bottle of beer.

As my pitiful flame continued, the cow started to shrink. First her right side returned to a normal appearance and then the left began to subside. Before she looked completely normal, the gas stopped coming. I wasn't unhappy to see the end of that flame, but there was still gas inside the cow that had to be removed. I moved the tube back and forth through the speculum until the smell of rumen gas told me that the end of the tube was back into the trapped air. After three or four manoeuvres like this and a little pushing on the cow's side by Mike, we had a perfectly normal-looking animal.

I pulled the tube up out of the cow's stomach through the

esophagus and out of the speculum. The position I had taken holding the cow's head had resulted in slimy saliva running down the insides of my coverall sleeves as far as my elbows. As I wiped my hands and arms off in the grass, Ingrid gathered up the equipment and was soon washing it off in a bucket of warm, soapy water.

The ease with which the gas had escaped through the tube made me think that this was an obstructive bloat, but just in case froth was involved, some preventative treatment was in order. I grabbed a bottle of anti-frothing agent from the truck and soon had it dispatched down the cow's gullet.

After washing my hands in Ingrid's bucket and taking off my slimy coveralls, I pulled my bill book from the front seat and walked over to Mike and Darryl.

"She should be fine now, Mike. Can you think of anything she might have eaten that would get stuck in her throat? Maybe carrots or apples?"

"No, all she eats is grass. I never gives her anything else."

As often happens, this seemed to have been a chance happening with no real lessons to learn and nothing for the owner to change in the way he looked after his cow.

As I wrote out the bill, I could hear Ingrid behind me snickering and trying to keep from breaking into laughter. When Mike and Darryl left to get some money from the house, Ingrid gave up her attempts at maintaining composure and laughed out loud.

"What's so funny?" I asked her.

She stopped long enough to get out, "Didn't you see his face?"

The two men returned with payment, and I checked out their faces. Mike looked fine, but Darryl was missing his eyebrows and had unusually short hair across the top of his forehead.

It was hard to be sympathetic.

6. The Eye of the Beholder

AS IN MANY NEWFOUNDLAND TOWNS, Carbonear has a Water Street running along the edge of the ocean. It starts at the bottom of the harbour and continues along the north side of the water. The portion of the road nearest the bottom of the harbour constituted the business section of town. The usual bank, post office and cenotaph shared this area with a variety of businesses. This was downtown small town at its best. Life strolled through this section of Carbonear with very occasional moments of excitement, like a building catching fire or a moose taking to the streets after a swim in the harbour.

The business district gradually thinned out as Water Street climbed a long, slow hill and died at the top, right at the funeral home. Coming down the other side, the street was lined with maples that nearly touched over the centre of the road. It was in this part of town that we had found our first home in Newfoundland. It didn't take long for the neighbours to learn that a vet was living in the area. My job was looking after the farm animals in my practice, but soon the dogs and cats began to appear. We didn't have much equipment for a small-animal practice, but it was impossible to turn away neighbours with pets in trouble.

One Thursday night the doorbell rang as we were finishing supper. A worried woman came into the house with a small poodle under her arm. She had been walking through some trees with her dog when the animal suddenly started howling and pawing at its face.

We cleared away the dishes from the kitchen table and gave the surface a wipe with a wet cloth. The hair around the poodle's left eye was matted with tears and the conjunctiva was red. A piece of wood about as big around as a pencil protruded from the corner of the eye socket.

I talked to the dog for a while and patted his head. It looked as though he had run into a stick during the walk in the woods. Once the poodle was calm, I'd easily be able to pull the stick out.

I tried catching the end of the stick with my fingers, but it was very short and slippery from tears. The next step was to use a pair of forceps. Working that close to the eyeball of a lively animal was going to be delicate work. A quick movement of the dog's head could give him another nasty poke.

First I asked the owner, "Would you mind holding your dog's head still while I pull that out?"

"I can't do that, I might hurt him! You're not going to hurt him, are you?"

I suggested that she might be more comfortable in the living room while Ingrid and I fixed up her dog. She agreed.

Ingrid was always reliable help when I worked with animals. I knew that if she held the dog's head, there would be no trouble from its teeth.

As Ingrid put her fingers around the dog's jaws and her arm around its neck, I attached the forceps to the stick and gave a little tug. Nothing happened. How far could a stick be stuck in a little dog's eye?

"Let's try this again. Hang on tight."

I pulled hard. The three-inch-long stick that came free must have been twisted around the eyeball and lodged against the very back of the socket.

Ingrid looked disturbed. "That was gross. I've got to get out of here." She left in a hurry.

When we talked about the case later, she said it wouldn't bother her at all to take a stick like that out of a person's eye, but it was different with a poor little dog that couldn't tell us anything about what hurt or what it would like done.

It wasn't long before we were to have another demonstration of the fact that things you aren't used to are difficult to deal with.

In rural Newfoundland in the 1980s, ideas about security and privacy were much different than now. If I went to pick up Ingrid from a shift in Emergency, it wasn't uncommon for me to be invited inside the clinic to watch her at work.

Shortly after the stick-in-the-eye case, I found myself at the hospital waiting for Ingrid. The nurse told her that I was in the waiting room, and she came out and said that I might be interested in seeing a case she was working on.

Her patient was a slightly inebriated man in his late twenties who had come through a glass door the hard way. He was bleeding profusely and the left side of his face was a mess. His temple and much of the cheek on one side was peeled open.

Ingrid had already cleaned the wound and was ready to patch him up. "You'll find this interesting," she told me. "I'm going to use a subcuticular stitch."

"You tell him, lady—put in the tickelars," slurred the patient.

"Just sit back, close your eyes, and I'll have you back together in a jiffy."

"Okay, lady." He leaned his head back and was soon snoring. Thanks to his self-medication, little tranquilizer was required to put him into a state where he didn't care much about the stitches.

I watched with interest as Ingrid pulled the skin farther and farther into place with each stitch. While my conscious mind was fascinated with Ingrid's impressive work—the glass-crasher wasn't going to be left with much scarring to remember his fall by—an unconscious rebellion was starting up. By the time she had six stitches in, I couldn't take any more.

"I've got to get out of here." I bolted for the waiting room. Despite my academic interest in the procedure, I found myself in a cold sweat and feeling woozy.

When Ingrid finished her work, she found me out in the waiting room reading a year-old copy of *Elle* magazine.

"You okay?"

"I'm fine," I heard myself say. "It wouldn't have bothered me if that was a dog or a cow with its face cut open. But a person? I can't imagine how you can do that."

7. Our House

WE WERE VERY HAPPY with our bright yellow house in Carbonear. We were directly across the road from a quiet playground on a lazy street tunnelled by maples. Since my employer, the provincial government, had paid for our move from Ontario, we had enough furniture to make parts of the house look lived in. The living room was graced by a rug we had been given for Christmas and an old couch donated by Ingrid's parents. The picture on our dysfunctional black-and-white television failed to fill the screen, but we didn't have much time to watch it anyway.

One of our great joys was to explore the surrounding area on foot. The road between Carbonear and a nearby fishing village called Freshwater was a twisting trail directly above the ocean. The rocky cliffs at the edge of the road fell off starkly to the water, interrupted only occasionally by minia-ture beaches of gravel. The magnificent vista from the road was punctuated by a number of islands. Tucker's Mill was a small outspearing of granite, stubbornly rising from the sea, that oddly resembled the map of Newfoundland. Maiden Island, with its swarms of terns, sat guarding the village just offshore, and Carbonear Island dominated the view. We had heard that when the French had conquered this part of

Newfoundland in the late 1600s, the locals moved to the island. Their resistance made Carbonear Island an impenetrable fortress. The first time we walked up over the final small hill that leads into Freshwater—a village surrounding a stark outcropping of rock—the sight astonished us. Houses lined the meandering shore and continued in and around this dominating granite structure, called locally "the tolt." A large white wooden church overlooked the community, its boat-filled harbour and its wharf. This was the place that we had dreamed of when we'd thought of moving to Newfoundland.

As we walked through the village, one building caught our eye: a dilapidated saltbox-style house sitting on the shore below the church. As we stopped in front of the house, the woman from next door stepped outside.

"Yoohoo, hello there! You're strange here, aren't ya?"

"Hi there. We were just walking through and admiring this old house."

"Bet you want to buy it and fix it up, don't ya?"

"Well, it is lovely." Ingrid and I looked at each other, knowing what we both were thinking.

"You can forget it. There have been hundreds of people looking at that old place and Uncle Alex will never sell it. That'll rot and fall down before that crowd can agree to let it go."

We spoke more about the house and found out that the owner was an elderly man who had moved to Carbonear, where he ran a small general store just down the road from our place. Ingrid said, "I'm going to see him and I'm going to convince him to sell that house to us."

For the next three weeks, every day after her shift, Ingrid stopped in at the general store where Uncle Alex worked. She asked him at the very first visit if he would like to sell his house in Freshwater. I think Uncle Alex liked having a cute young woman drop in to see him, and he did nothing to discourage Ingrid's visits. Every time she went by the store they would talk about the house. After two weeks, he allowed that it might be time to sell the place if his relatives would agree.

Ingrid arrived home one night with an excited grin on her face. "Uncle Alex has agreed to show us the house!"

After work the next day we practically skipped down the road to the store. Uncle Alex was sitting on a stool at his usual station by the checkout counter. When we entered he leaned forward and spat a viscid wad into the tobacco tin settled by his foot. He wiped his wrist across the stain that ran from the corner of his mouth and looked up with watery eyes. He held our gaze for what seemed like minutes and then wordlessly gave us a quick nod. We both understood that we were part of a secret conspiracy that could not be spoken of while there were customers in the store.

Ingrid and I walked to the back of the shop and took in the questionable vegetables, the swarms of flies, buckets of salt meat and rows of cans of Vienna sausages. There was no point talking with Uncle Alex until the store was empty.

When the last customer left, Uncle Alex stood, walked to the door and looked out suspiciously in both directions. Then he locked the door and returned to his stool. Ingrid and I went back to the counter and stood like the two supplicants that we were.

"So you want to see the old place, do ya?" Uncle Alex leaned forward and let another stream of tobacco juice fly into the can.

Ingrid was quick to answer. "Sure, that's great. We can get our car and drive you up to Freshwater, if you like."

"Now hold on, lady, don't you be in such a hurry. I'll drive. Let me get the keys for the house."

Uncle Alex walked back through the store and out a small door in the rear. He always slurred his words when he spoke, but it concerned me that his travel across the store could hardly be described as a straight line. We sat down on two chairs and waited.

It was at least fifteen minutes before Uncle Alex returned— a long time to fetch a set of keys.

"Wait here just a minute." Uncle Alex repeated his furtive glances out the front door. "Come on, let's get in the car."

With all of this apparent secrecy around the trip to Freshwater, I expected us to roar out of his garage and be off to the village before anyone could see us. But instead, the car crept out of the garage and turned down the road toward the village. The highest speed we achieved was around twelve miles an hour. Our progress was further hindered by Uncle Alex's need to spew out a jet of tobacco juice every few minutes. He would stop the car in the middle of his lane, open his door and lean low and far out into the road before spitting. Every time he did this, I worried that an oncoming car would take the door off and decapitate him.

We finally pulled up in front of the old house. Uncle Alex hauled himself out of the car and ambled unsteadily to the front door. He patted his jacket and pants and spat on the ground.

"I've forgotten the keys. We'll have to drive back to the store."

We were not keen on spending any more time than necessary in a car with Uncle Alex.

"That's fine, Uncle Alex," Ingrid told him. "You get the keys and we'll sit here and enjoy the sun."

As he drove away we stood on the front step and admired the scenery. The large open field across the road gave the property a feeling of spaciousness. I wondered who owned this land and hoped that no one would ever spoil the effect by putting a building there.

It was a beautiful day and we were happy to move around to the back and watch the sea. We found a spot between two lilac trees just over the ocean. Time did not exist for us while Uncle Alex drove to Carbonear and back.

The car inched its way down the hill from the big wooden church. From somewhere inside his rumpled jacket, Alex pulled an eight-inch-long set of cast-iron keys. With the door open at last, we all stepped inside.

The house was more than a hundred and thirty years old. A calendar on the wall indicated that no one had lived in the place for more than twenty years. The floor in the living room sagged over half a foot across its width. A bare wire ran across the ceiling to an ancient light bulb. The upstairs hall was transected by a rusting pipe just below head height that brought heat from the chimney to rooms across the hall. The house was on the ocean. It was perfect.

Ingrid could hardly contain her excitement. "If we had this place we could—"

"Now you just hold on now, missy," Uncle Alex interrupted. "I told you I'd *show* you the house. I didn't say I would *sell* it to you."

The two of us visibly slumped, worried that our joint enthusiasm had ruined our chances to own this wonderful spot.

Uncle Alex turned for the door. "We can talk about *that* tomorrow."

From past experience we knew that we could only talk to Uncle Alex after his store was closed and empty in the afternoon. The next day seemed to take forever. Finally the time came to visit Uncle Alex's store again.

We dropped in just before his regular closing time. As the last customer left, Alex went to the front door, checked that the coast was clear and flipped the lock. He came over to us and pulled a piece of paper from his shirt pocket.

"I have a number written here. This is the price of the house. There will be no arguing over this price."

The paper bore a very reasonable number written in a shaky hand. Ingrid and I grinned at each other.

"There are a couple of catches, though."

What now?

"First, you never tell anyone what that number is."

We nodded eagerly.

"Second, you have to take the field across the road."

We had our house.

8. Robert

FROM TIME TO TIME I was joined on my rounds by students seeking the work experience they needed in order to apply to veterinary school. Perhaps my favourite of all of these students was the first, Robert. Shortly after I arrived in Newfoundland, Robert's father became my new dentist, and we soon had an arrangement where I looked after his dogs in return for him looking after my teeth. When he told me that his oldest son, who was just finishing high school, was interested in becoming a vet, I said the boy was welcome to accompany me any time that he was free.

An early call we did together was an evening summons to the town of North River, where a cow was having trouble delivering her calf. During the forty-minute drive Robert asked whether anything like the stories in the James Herriot books ever happened to me.

I told him to stick around.

North River is set in a beautiful valley between two rocky ridges along a slow, winding river. Turning off the main road through Conception Bay north at Clarke's Beach, you can follow the waterway through the town. The scenery of the river and the hills had obviously attracted people with money to build large and beautiful houses throughout the valley.

The fancy houses tend to be not too far from the ocean and the main highway. As you drive down the road into North River the homes become more modest. Our destination was the second-last house.

I'd been given a good description of the place we were looking for, and we had no trouble picking it out. The fact that there were about a dozen trucks parked outside and the barn lights were on gave us an idea that something exciting was going on inside.

As we pulled up to the barn, Garfield, a thin man of about sixty-five with neatly combed hair, rushed out to greet us.

"I'm so glad you could come, Doctor. My cow's havin' trouble gettin' this calf out and this time I'm not lettin' the boys have a go at her. Last year my other cow couldn't calve by herself so me and the lads got some ropes on the calf's legs to help her along. Lost the cow and the calf both. Come on to the barn, sir, and have a look at me cow."

The barn was small and warm, not just from the two cows inside but also from the fifteen neighbours who filled the available space.

The owner beamed with pride as he escorted me through the barn door. "This is the vet, boys. I've paid to have him come and have a look at Princess."

I gathered that the price of a vet bill would be a major challenge to Garfield and he intended all of his neighbours to know what good care he took of his animals. It seemed no expense was too high for him to ensure Princess's health and contentment.

From the doorway I could see Princess arching her back at regular intervals and letting out grunts of discomfort.

"How long has she been pushing like this, Garfield?"

"Started about fifteen minutes before the wife called you."

This is information more usually obtained by phone before leaving on a call. In this case, all I'd heard by phone was panic-stricken wailing from Garfield's wife, who wasn't exactly sure what was happening or how long it had been going on, but relayed the message that I was to come at once to check on the cow.

Sometimes it is difficult to tell when a delivering cow is in trouble. Usually I don't worry too much until she has been pushing intermittently for about an hour or she lies down and constantly strains with no progress. By my calculations this cow was still in the normal range.

I returned to the truck to pull on my boots, fill a pail with warm water and squirt in a little disinfectant for good measure.

Robert and I climbed over the fence into the pen as the neighbours crowded in closer to see what would happen. There was a good chance that this would be a highlight of North River's social activity for the week.

Robert held Princess's tail to the side as I rolled up my right coverall sleeve and scrubbed my arm with the iodine-tinged water. Next, I cleaned the cow's vulva and perineal area before gently pushing my hand in. My arm was in as far as the elbow when I encountered something hard. With a little exploration I found two front legs pointing straight out at me with a nose following close behind.

This is the normal and easiest way that a calf can come out of a cow. The calf "dives" out as the cow pushes. Problems with deliveries come when the calf doesn't get into this diving position, instead coming backwards or sideways or having some part like a leg or head caught up behind the pelvis. If the calf is in the right position and the cow has a large enough birth canal for the calf to fit through and she is healthy, there usually isn't any trouble.

This calf was coming in a perfect position, there seemed to be plenty of room, and judging from her condition, the cow should have no trouble delivering the calf by herself.

With no rush to proceed with the delivery, this was an ideal opportunity to teach Robert a little about obstetrics.

"Would you mind if Robert here had a feel at your cow?" I asked Garfield. "He's a student who wants to be a vet."

"Yes sir, you go right ahead now. If this young fella can learn something from Princess while you cure her, that would be wonderful."

Robert and I changed positions and he rolled up his sleeve and washed his arm. My student certainly looked the vet part as he prepared to examine Princess.

Under his breath Robert confided, "This is great—I've never seen anything born before." As I directed, he washed off the back of the cow, coned his fingers and thumb together and gently entered the birth passage. Just before his elbow would have disappeared, his eyes grew even wider. "I feel something," he loudly whispered. A few snickers came from the audience.

"What do you think you have there?" I asked.

"It's the head."

From the position of his arm I could tell that he couldn't be in far enough to reach the head, so I suggested, "Feel around and make sure it's the head."

After a few seconds of hard concentration, Robert said to me, "It's a foot. I can feel the leg coming from behind it."

Without having the experience of feeling a calf inside a cow, it is difficult to imagine how anyone could confuse a head and a hoof. But this type of examination is much more difficult than it seems. Few things we do in everyday life can prepare us for an exploration that involves the sense of touch without using our sight. We take for granted that we can pick things out by their feel, but usually it is sight that gives us the bulk of our useful information. Robert was reminding me how lost and hopeless I felt the first few times I did internal examinations on cattle.

"Move around a bit more inside and see what else you can feel," I told him. "You should be able to find the head and distinguish the nose and eyes."

Robert slowly inched his way in, and from his expression I could tell that he was discovering new worlds with every movement of his hand. It's hard to describe the thrill of first feeling and recognizing a live animal and then sensing it move before it is born.

Sometime around when Robert's shoulder looked to be in danger of disappearing, the extra mass inside of Princess started to irritate her. She turned her head back, let out a disapproving bawl and arched her back. With the effort she loosed a stream of watery manure down the back of Robert's coveralls. Robert, undeterred, looked at me, and in a voice not intended for the crowd, said, "Just watch—next time she'll do it in my face." The approving roars from the onlookers told us he had misjudged his volume.

Because everything was progressing normally, ordinarily I would have left poor Princess to herself and let her get on with the calving. Still, I could see that if I left now, Garfield would feel that the vet never did what he'd called him for, and there was always the chance that I could drive all the way home only to hear that something had gone wrong and a second visit would be needed. As well, this was a chance for Robert to see his first animal born.

From the back of the truck I picked out two stainless steel chains and the pulling handles that hooked into them. Trying to pull out an uncooperative calf with bare hands is frustrating work, as its legs are too slippery and slimy to get any kind of grip on. While ropes may look less like torture instruments than chains, they have the disadvantage of continuing to tighten as they are pulled on. The links in the chains catch on themselves, so chains don't tighten and cut the calf's skin.

The real work of most deliveries is getting the calf into the right position and putting the chains onto the parts you decide to pull on. This one was easy. I disinfected the chains, reached inside and put a loop above and a half hitch below the fetlock of both feet. It was now a matter of a little tug on the legs and making sure that the head continued to follow in line.

I decided that it would make most sense for me to guide the head along as someone else pulled on the chains.

"Do you mind if the student pulls out the calf?" I asked Garfield.

"That would be great!" He beamed at the audience in the barn. This was turning into a real event. For a few days Garfield would be a local celebrity.

I snugged the handles onto the chains and passed them to Robert. "When you see her starting into a contraction, give a little pull and see if you can move the calf ahead a little. I'll keep my arm in here and make sure that everything is coming the right way."

Princess pushed and let out a little groan. Robert planted his feet and leaned back on the chains. From inside I could feel the head come forward a few inches.

"That's great. A few more like that and we'll have a calf."

The crowd was on their feet and pressing in around the pen to see the new calf arrive. The mumbles, hacks and coughs that had punctuated the proceedings thus far all gave way to an expectant silence.

Princess pushed again, Robert pulled, and the calf's nose came into view. My part of the process was done, so I sat back on a bale of hay to watch Robert's first delivery.

The next contraction brought the calf out past its shoulders.

This was obviously a time of great discomfort for poor Princess. She let out a deafening bawl, turned to look at Robert and arched her back. There was way too much pressure on her, and something had to give.

I don't really think that she looked back in order to take aim, but she might as well have, considering the accuracy of the stream of diarrhea that followed. The mess hit Robert directly in his face.

The neighbours howled and slapped each other on the backs. One fellow even fell to the ground from the general sense of hilarity.

Robert seemed not to notice. He reached up with his fingers to wipe the outside and inside of his glasses, and as soon as he could see he gave one last pull that brought the calf onto the sawdust.

He helped take the chains off the legs and watched in wonder as the calf shook his head, blew the slime out of his nose and blinked his eyes. I never tire of the beauty of the first few seconds of life. It is one of the great joys of my work.

This job wasn't quite done, as we still had to attend to the cow and calf. First I reached back inside the cow to make sure that no damage was done or a second calf was waiting to come out. Everything was perfect. While Robert washed off the chains I fetched an injection of oxytocin to help shrink down the cow's uterus and some iodine to disinfect the calf's navel. I showed Robert where the injection and the iodine went and he finished up our job.

The spectators headed back to their trucks and the night filled with the sound of ignitions. Headlights spun through the air as the trucks turned onto the road. By the time we had everything returned to the truck we were alone with Garfield.

"Come in now and we'll get you some money and a cup of tea."

We followed him into the house and sat down at the kitchen table. After I made out the bill, Garfield's wife brought me full payment for the night's work and a cup of tea and fresh homemade bread. The happiness that Garfield gained from his healthy cow and new calf and that Robert had from his first delivery added to the warmth of the surroundings.

A few slices of bread and a couple of stories later we said our goodbyes and set off for home in the truck.

I turned to my young assistant. "Do you remember how you asked me if anything like James Herriot stories ever happens on my calls?"

9. A Difficult Man

SOMETIME DURING MY FIRST YEAR of work, my boss asked me if I would be interested in coming along with him to see a chicken barn in Carbonear. The position of provincial veterinarian involved supervising the seven regional veterinarians (of which I was one) and developing and maintaining government policy that related to animal health. Doc Smith, the first provincial veterinarian during my time in practice, also looked after most of the poultry work in the province. Being in practice alone, I jumped at every opportunity to work with another vet.

This was my first visit to Samuel, one of the most unpleasant people I have ever met. No sooner had we entered the barn than he started complaining about how long it had taken us to come. With this out of the way, he started asking why I had come along. It was obvious to him that I didn't know anything about chickens and it was a waste of government money to have me on this call. I hadn't even been introduced.

The problem was that too many of his young chicks were dying. It didn't take Doc Smith and me long to see what the cause was. The feeders for the chicks were set too high and they couldn't reach in to eat. Quick post-mortems on a few chicks showed that none of them had any food in their stomachs. This was a basic blunder that no serious chicken farmer should make. Sam grumbled through the visit and insisted that something else must be killing his chicks. He kept muttering that neither of us knew anything. Despite our simple and obvious diagnosis, he insisted we were wrong and that his problems could be solved only with antibiotics. It seemed to me that the only reason Sam had called us was that we had access to drugs he felt he needed.

As we walked back to the truck, I asked Doc if Samuel was always this difficult. Doc Smith was a gentleman. He came from a different era, when politeness, good manners and proper dress were expected. He wore a white shirt and tie under his coveralls to every call, and I don't remember him ever having a negative comment about anyone. I wondered if Sam would test his limits.

"You could call him difficult, and he isn't the best chicken farmer we have. The last time I was called to see him he had a floor full of drowned birds. It turned out that he stopped in to look at the barn on the way to a dance and when he saw the waterers leaking he just turned off the lights and closed the door. That's not good farming."

It wasn't long until I had to deal with Samuel again, and this time alone. I had just settled into dinner one evening when the phone rang. Sam's daughter was in a panic. She'd had a horse down for a couple of hours with a swollen face and she didn't know what to do. It was always frustrating when people with sick animals waited until after the office closed to call in. I had driven by their place on my way home after work. Still, this sounded important, so I said I would be there as soon as I could. Dinner would be reheated and eaten alone that night.

As I drove up to Sam's house, I could see him standing in the driveway. Despite my initial impression of the man, I tried a friendly approach.

I rolled down the window as I drove up the drive. "Sounds like you've got some trouble today, Sam."

His answer surprised me. "What the hell are you doing here?"

I explained that his daughter had called and that it sounded like he had a bit of an emergency on his hands.

"You don't come here unless I call you." The simplest solution would have been to smile and tell him he was right; I wouldn't come to his farm again under any conditions unless he called me first. But to walk away from this kind of bullying wasn't in my nature. There were two issues here. I had been called away from a meal at home to do this call, and there was quite possibly an animal that needed help.

"Tell you what, Sam. I've been called out here to see your horse, so this is a call. It's up to you whether you want me to look at the horse, but either way you're getting a bill for this visit."

He started cursing me and letting me know exactly what he thought of my qualities as a vet and as a human being.

"Hold on, Sam. Do you want your horse seen?"

"Of course not, you idiot."

"Okay, I've got something for you." I reached across the front seat of the truck for my pile of invoices and picked up a pen. As calmly as I could, I wrote out a bill for an emergency visit, with no time added for an examination. "Here, this is yours." I handed him the bill and drove out his driveway.

It was a couple of years before I saw Sam again. One morning I decided to go in to the office early to finish some paperwork and catch up on a few things in the lab. On days like this, I would leave the door to the office unlocked so that any farmers who came in early wouldn't have to wait outside for opening time.

Samuel burst in through the door. "I'm in a rush, get me some penicillin."

"What do you need it for, Sam?"

"My racehorse. She pulled a muscle last night and I need some penicillin."

"Sorry, Sam, but there are a couple of problems here. First off, penicillin isn't any good for pulled muscles. Second, you owe us money for a couple of previous calls. I've been told not to give service to you until those bills are paid."

"I don't care about that, just get me the damn penicillin."

"Let me explain again. Before you can get anything here you have to pay your bills. Then, when your bills are paid, we will sell you drugs for problems that the drugs will work on. This isn't a grocery store for drugs."

"You useless son of a bitch." Sam strode over to the fire extinguisher hanging on the wall. "I'd like to smash your head in with this thing." He looked up and down the fire extinguisher before turning for the exit. "Before this day is done, you are gonna be in big trouble."

"Always a pleasure to see you, Sam. Drop in any time you'd like to have a chat."

Mumbling curses, he flung the door open with such force that it crashed against the wall.

I had no doubt that Sam wasn't bluffing with his threat of causing grief for me. Right away I phoned my boss's office in St. John's and let him know what had happened. It wouldn't surprise me if a trumped-up complaint came in, and I wanted to pre-empt this possibility with my version of events.

As my colleagues came into the office I related the morning's adventure. No one was too surprised, as they had all had dealings with Samuel and all knew how he behaved. You had to give Samuel credit for one thing. He did treat everyone the same.

About an hour after opening time, Samuel appeared back in the office. First he marched into the office next to mine, where the local agricultural representative, Blake, worked. I heard him ask for penicillin and then I heard Blake say that only the vet could sell drugs in this office. Sam stormed out of the office and turned to Sharon.

"Get me a bottle of penicillin."

"I'm sorry, Samuel, but you know that only the vet can give you penicillin."

"That son of a bitch. I've had about enough of this. I'm going home and phoning your boss in St. John's about this."

Putting down the surgery book I was looking through in my office, I called out to my disgruntled client. "Sam, don't run off yet. We'll save you some time. Sharon, call the office in St. John's and give the phone to this gentleman."

Sharon dialed our main office and handed the receiver to Sam.

"Hello, is this the vet office in St. John's? Are you in charge? I came in to see your vet out here and he refuses to come out to see a horse I have down with pneumonia."

Even Samuel had outdone himself with this outlandish lie. While I couldn't hear what my boss was saying on the phone, I knew that he understood what was happening and it was easy to fill in his side of the conversation.

"That's right, pneumonia ... Whaddaya mean, unpaid bills? You son of a bitch!" He threw the receiver down on the desk and took three steps that put him in the doorway of my office. "I'd just love to punch you right in the mouth."

I had never had a client—or anyone—threaten me in quite that way before. For a second I wondered what to do. Just as in previous encounters with this man, I decided that backing away from his behaviour would only make things worse.

I slid my chair back from the desk and stood. I took a few steps to the doorway of the office and stood so my nose nearly touched his.

"Okay, Sam, here's your chance. Why don't you take a smack at me? I suggest you hit me pretty hard. When you're done, there are two things I might do. I may go upstairs and talk to the lawyer that works up there, or I may hit you back hard enough that you won't get up for a week."

I'm not sure whether these words coming from my mouth were more of a surprise to Sam or to me. I have always avoided confrontation and I hate fights in any form. But the bravado did its work. Sam walked quickly out of the office. It was obvious that the battle—and likely the war—was mine.

My boss phoned later in the day. He would be notifying Sam that he wasn't to enter our office again and that the staff would call the police if he ever did. The support was appreciated, but it wasn't really needed. That was the last time I ever laid eyes on the man.

10. Pogo the Cow Herder

MY CONSTANT COMPANION and friend after my first year of work was Pogo. With a green eye, a blue eye, no tail and every colour of brown imaginable in her coat, she was not an ordinary-looking dog.

In our home village of Freshwater, cows, horses and goats were free to roam. Most people kept their lawns and steps clean with a fence. We never seemed to find time to build one. Our solution to the roaming animals was an Australian shepherd.

Dogs of that breed are natural herders, and Pogo's greatest passion in life was chasing cows. Two or three times a week during the summer months, the Freshwater cattle would decide to check out the availability of grass in our corner of the village. Once they got within fifty yards of our house, Pogo would run from window to window whining to be let out. Once outside, she would tear down the road, herd the cows into a group and hustle them away.

Pogo made it look easy. We discovered how much skill herding required when the neighbour's dog decided to help. The cows came in close to our house and Pogo started putting the animals into one tight group. She would run a quick circle around them and gradually tighten her radius. Once she had the herd in a configuration she liked, she would start them moving.

The neighbour's dog watched, and thinking this looked like great fun, raced over and confronted one of the cows face to face. I could almost see Pogo rolling her eyes at this show of ineptitude. Everyone knows that cows are attacked at the heels.

Pogo nipped at one cow's back legs and got her moving. The second dog watched and tried to copy Pogo's methods. The novice herder went behind another cow and gingerly bit at its heels. The resulting kick was almost too fast to see and it sent the shocked animal about ten feet through the air and then rolling along the grass. The dog rose, shook herself and limped away with a clearer appreciation of the skills the job required.

During working hours, Pogo travelled with me in the truck. No matter what else was happening or whatever the time of day or night, she was keen to go. Her usual role was just to watch scenery while we drove and wait in the truck during calls. On long drives we had lengthy conversations as she rested her head on my lap. Occasionally she had more exciting work.

One hot and humid August day, I was called to the Cape Shore to examine a lame bull and some calves with diarrhea. After dealing with the calves, I set off with Pogo and the community pasture manager, Dermot, to look at the bull.

I have never really understood why an enormous animal would allow itself to be chased and herded by a person six to eight times smaller. Apparently, the bull never really understood this either. No amount of yelling, jumping up and down, threatening or prodding with sticks would get him to budge. Soon, however, we found his weak spot and had the bull chasing a half-dozen attractive cows in front of him.

The reason for all this chasing was to lead the bull out onto the road and then about a quarter of a mile to a pen with restraining facilities. Since this type of work was Pogo's specialty, I suggested to Dermot that he drive my truck down to the pen while the dog and I brought the cattle down. It took little coaxing for Pogo to run over to the group, separate out a few cows and start moving them. Soon, though, it became apparent that there had been a serious flaw in my dog's herding education. It was simple enough to get her to chase cattle, but I found out that I had no say in the question of which direction they should be chased.

Of course Pogo soon had the cows running at a furious pace—but going the wrong way. The dog was easy enough to stop, but the cows were another matter. I decided the best approach to the situation was to run past the cows and chase them back. Unfortunately, the road was narrow, and the cows mistook my effort at passing them for further chasing. To add to the frustration of trying to outrun a group of cows on a hot day while wearing boots and coveralls, Pogo sauntered up alongside me with a self-satisfied grin looking for praise. In the heat of the moment it seemed to me that the only appropriate response was to apply a boot to the dog's back end. I've seen dozens of cows lash out at Pogo with deadly hooves and I don't recall ever seeing her hit. It must have been simple work for her to avoid my feeble footwork.

The kick put me off balance and I was soon down on the gravel with skinned hands and knees and feelings of foolishness and guilt.

Perhaps it was a quarter of a mile or more up the road when I finally passed the cows and managed to turn them around. The chase back to the pen, where the pasture manager was waiting, was uneventful. Pogo saw the open gate to the side of the road and expertly steered the animals in. The manager, who seemed to notice nothing unusual about the length of time it had taken us to bring the cows down, commented on what a good herder the dog was. Too exhausted to reply, I started to work on the bull while Pogo sat proudly by, satisfied with a job well done.

Dermot had invited me to stop in at his place in St. Bride's before the two-and-a-half-hour journey home and was waiting for me as I pulled into his driveway.

"Bring the dog in. She did great work today, I'm sure she'd love to come inside."

Pogo was thrilled and sat proudly by my side when we settled in the house.

Dermot turned to his wife. "Maid, put on a cup of tea for the vet. Send the young fella up to the shop for something for a sandwich."

Dermot's son jumped up from his seat and ran out of the house. He was back in five minutes and handed a can of processed meat to his father. Dermot's wife poured cups of hot water with individual tea bags and set out a can of Carnation milk and a bowl of sugar. Dermot snapped the key off the meat tin and started winding open the can. Once the lid was off, he slid the contents out of the container and onto the lid.

"Do you mind if I gives the dog a little slice of meat? She worked hard today."

I wasn't really sure that Pogo had earned any meat with her antics that day, but I agreed. "Just give her a little bit so she doesn't throw up in the truck."

"That'll be fine. Come here, doggie."

Clarence snapped open his pocket knife and cut a thin slice of meat for Pogo. The dog looked up at me, stretched and cautiously approached Dermot's chair. As Dermot held out his right hand—the one holding the dog's reward—Pogo dove at his left, grabbing and swallowing the main hunk of meat.

The room went silent. Pogo turned, swaggered back to my chair and sat licking her lips. The dog had eaten everyone's snacks at a single bound. I sat back and waited for a reaction.

Dermot looked back and forth from the empty lid to the remaining sliver of meat. His wife's eyes were wide with surprise and her hand moved up in front of her mouth.

Dermot broke the uncomfortable spell as he tossed the empty lid onto the table, slapped his hand on his knee and roared with laughter.

"That's some clever dog, maid. Get us some bakeapple jam for this bread."

I would take homemade jam on fresh-baked bread over processed meat any day, and Pogo could forget about having any.

11. You Knew Just Exactly

EVERYONE LOVES CREDIT for a job well done. When we work hard and everything goes right, it is human nature to enjoy a well-deserved thank you. But credit doesn't always come when it should. Sometimes no one seems to appreciate our best efforts. Other times, the effusive praise and credit we receive don't make any sense at all.

Randy lived in the hollow between Carbonear and Victoria. His house and barn were set just off the road with a few other houses. He had called the office first thing one Thursday morning.

"Doc, I don't like the look of me cow."

"What do you think is wrong with her?"

"Now, it seems to me her elder is terrible gathered up."

"How long has she been like this?"

"Can't rightly say, but it strikes me she hasn't been right for a nice while."

"Will you be in this morning?"

"Well, I have to drive Mudder up to the hospital for some tests and then I have to move some nets down from the wharf."

"Will you be home by one?"

"Oh, I would say I likely will."

"I'll see you at one, then."

A little explanation may be in order. An "elder" is an udder and "gathered up" usually means infected, but it can also mean swollen, red or just about anything else that can be wrong with any part of an animal.

I had a horse castration down the bay, so Randy's opening in his calendar at one fit my schedule quite nicely. While the horse might not have agreed, I felt the castration went very well and I had time to get home for a sandwich before heading out to Randy's.

Feeling full and somewhat sluggish after my noon break, I pulled the truck up beside Randy's barn. I hopped over the little stream that ran between the barn and the road, walked around the building and went in the back door.

Randy was chewing on a straw and leaning with one arm over the back end of a cow. He didn't seem to be in a hurry to do much else. Like every other time I saw Randy, he was dressed in barn clothes: three or four layers of jackets, sweaters and shirts overlaid with a wide pair of suspenders holding up a very loose pair of pants. His long, full beard, slightly portly constitution and slow manner of movement and speech gave him an ageless demeanour. I always figured that he was somewhere between his late thirties and early nineties.

He took the straw from his mouth. "You made it up."

"I did. Is this our patient?"

"This is Mol. She really doesn't seem right."

Mol was a Jersey, a breed of light brown dairy cow that was a bit of a rarity in our area. Jerseys are normally quite thin, and sometimes in the winter in rural Newfoundland they are a little thinner than they should be. Randy, however, was a conscientious farmer and his cattle were always clean and in the best of shape. Mol looked too thin for one of Randy's cows, and her eyes had that listless look of a sick animal.

After a quick check-over, I moved to Mol's side to have a look at her udder.

Between her back legs where there should normally be a soft, pliable pendulation of flesh, I found a hard, dark piece of tissue. The udder was cold and stiff, with a colour that ran from dark blue to black. The skin looked like cardboard and was peeling away in a manner that suggested some gross exaggeration of a sunburn. The way that Mol stood with her back legs tenderly spread indicated that this was a painful condition.

Infection of the udder, or mastitis, is one of the most commonly seen problems in dairy cows. These animals have been bred over the centuries to make milk, and lots of it. A modern dairy cow can produce more than eight gallons of milk a day, or over two thousand, five hundred gallons in a year, far beyond what they naturally need to produce to feed their calves. The extra milk, of course, is the reason that dairy farms are so successful at providing the milk that we drink. But this extra production comes at a cost to the cow. In order to be economically useful, a cow must produce milk at a level that puts great strain on her body. Dairy cows commonly run into health problems caused by this unnaturally high production of milk.

Mastitis is the result of micro-organisms getting into the milk either from the inside of the cow or, more commonly, from the environment. A small amount of dirt carried up through the teat can start an infection in the udder. If mastitis is seen early enough, it can usually be cured by a combination of removing milk from the udder and introducing an antibiotic up through the teat opening. In most cases, the antibiotic kills the offending bacteria. The antibiotic-tainted milk is then removed from the cow and with any luck she can come back into normal milk production. Mol's case was about as bad as mastitis gets. Her whole udder was either dead or dying. There was no chance that she would ever produce any milk again. The future didn't look good for Mol.

"Randy, I'm not very happy with the way Mol is looking. That udder on her is so bad that her milking days are over."

"So what do we do with her, Doc?"

"I guess the reason you have Mol is for her milk, and she won't be giving you any more of that, so maybe the best thing would be to put her down."

There was a long pause. "Well you see, Doc, Mol has been awfully good to us, so I really can't see doing that to her. I could keep her around. She's earned a bit more hay and feed."

"We can try, Randy, but I can't make any promises. She's really sick, and even with treatment she may die on us."

"Well, you just do what you can, Doc."

Cows with gangrenous mastitis this far advanced often don't survive, but I was willing to try with Mol. I thought our best option would be to amputate the whole udder. This was a major operation I'd never done before and I didn't relish the idea of getting into surgery that was over my head. Because a dairy cow produces such great amounts of milk, huge blood vessels supply the udder. A full amputation means cutting through these arteries and veins and tying them off before the cow bleeds to death.

I didn't have the nerve to try the surgery right there, and besides, I hoped that some time with antibiotic in Mol's system would improve her chances of surviving the surgery.

"I'll be back in a minute, Randy."

I walked back around the barn and over the stream to my truck, wondering what I was getting myself into. From the back of the truck, I picked out a bottle of antibiotic, some anti-inflammatory medication and a tube of skin ointment.

Back in the barn, Mol got a syringe full of antibiotic into the hip muscles and another with the anti-inflammatory into her jugular vein. I left Randy with the rest of the bottle of antibiotic to inject once a day and the ointment to rub into the skin at the edges of the dead udder.

At home that night, I read up on udder amputation. It didn't sound much better than I remembered it from school. It was a bloody procedure requiring equipment and a surgery suite I just didn't have. This was a problem I often ran into. Alone in practice in a rural setting, I was expected to deal with everything that came up by myself. Books could talk about referring cases to universities or surgical centres, but the realities of my practice meant that whatever was going to be done, I would have to do alone.

I often drove by Randy's barn on my way home from calls. The next day on my way home for a late supper, as I approached the turnoff to his barn I wondered if I should stop in to see how Mol was doing. No, this wouldn't help anything; she had all the drugs she needed to improve, and besides, I was hungry.

The weekend came next and I spent a lot of Saturday and Sunday wondering about how I would ever do this surgery.

Monday, I drove past Randy's again, and again I didn't drop in.

Tuesday's and Wednesday's calls took me in a different direction, and I tried to persuade myself that more time with the antibiotic inside her would help Mol with the operation. But I knew I was just procrastinating.

Thursday morning I decided it was time for action. I called Randy.

"Hi, Randy, how are things?"

"Oh, not so bad."

"How's Mol?"

"Oh, not so bad."

"Are you going to be around today?"

"Well, I was just getting ready to take Mudder to the hospital and then I have to help some fellers take a motor off a boat down by the wharf . . ."

"Will you be home by one?"

"Oh, I would say I likely will."

Despite my feelings of being stuck in some kind of a time warp, I was filled with both dread and relief at the prospect of getting back to Mol. The morning's calls were routine, and most of the time the back of my head was filled with visions of the upcoming surgery.

At one o'clock I drove back to Randy's farm. I collected my surgical tools and went into the barn. Randy was standing in exactly the same position he had been in when I'd dropped in a week earlier. Looking at him leaning on the cow with the straw in his mouth, I wondered whether he had even moved in the last week.

Mol looked a little brighter; the antibiotics had done some good. Her eyes looked better and she was chewing a little mouthful of hay.

I bent down to examine the udder. The tissue death I had seen the week before had progressed in the affected area, but the disease had not moved farther into the cow. Closer examination showed that the udder was actually separating from the body and was hanging by bits of leathery dead skin. It was now completely black and oozed foul-smelling pus and clear fluid.

Before beginning the amputation, I thought I would just take a little cut at some of the supporting skin to see what would happen. I sliced my scalpel through the dead skin that ran along the edge of the udder—and the entire udder fell off the cow and landed on the ground with a sickening thud. Mol didn't flinch, and there was no bleeding.

Randy looked over my shoulder. "My son, you knew just exactly when to come back, didn't you?"

I shrugged and turned away to hide my guilty smile.

Randy scooped up the udder with a shovel and shook his head as he left the barn. "My sonny boy," he muttered to himself in disbelief.

I left with my reputation undeservedly inflated.

12. Totalling the Truck

BACK WHEN I FIRST MOVED to Newfoundland, my first boss, Doc Smith, had warned me that the weather could be bad in the winter and the roads could be treacherous. I was still young and invincible and didn't worry much. After all, I had been raised and learned to drive in the wilds of northern Ontario. My childhood was spent in Kapuskasing, where temperatures dipped down to forty below and conditions were considered harsh enough for a major car manufacturer to set up a cold-weather testing station.

At three o'clock one morning the phone went off like a bomb. I bolted upright with a pounding heart. Where was I? What was that noise? The second ring of the phone sounded just like a phone, and I gathered my composure as I picked up the receiver.

"Yeah?"

"How are ya, Doc?"

"I'm great. How are you?"

"I'm good but the cow's not. You'd better come right now."

"What's the trouble?"

"She's been pushin' since just before midnight and nothin's comin'."

It was another calving. It seemed there were a lot of them coming in lately.

"I'll be right there. Who's this calling?" I thought this information might be helpful in getting me to the cow.

"It's me. Obe."

"Great, Obe. I'll be there as soon as I can."

Obe Milford had a farm about an hour away on a stretch of road called Roaches Line. He lived by himself with his twenty Charolais cattle and didn't call the vet unless things were bad. Obe's calls were always serious.

Ingrid rolled over in bed. "What was that?"

"I've got to go deliver a calf. Go back to sleep."

"I think I *am* sleeping."

Pogo's response was quite different. She knew and loved the routine for calls in the middle of the night. As soon as the phone rang and the light went on in our room, she would station herself by the front door. There was no way she was going to miss a ride somewhere exciting just because it was three o'clock in the morning. One of the joys of having a dog is how easy it is to amuse them. Pogo let you know that nothing in the world was more exciting than going somewhere in the truck.

Like Pogo, I had a routine for night calls. As I dressed, I would mutter to myself about how normal people with normal jobs didn't have to work at unreasonable hours like this. If the drive was long, I'd pack an apple and a couple of cookies to sustain me through the trip. After a quick glass of water, I'd grab my keys and head out to the truck.

I paused before getting in the truck to look around Freshwater and up into the sky. There had been rain earlier in the evening, and though it was winter, it was warm enough that the pavement was wet and not icy. Only a few lights were visible around the village, and the stars shone as they only can out in the country. This wasn't so bad. This was going to be an adventure. Like every other time I went out on night calls, I came around to Pogo's view of the proceedings.

As the dog and I pulled away from the house, I switched on the radio and tuned in to CBC, which tended to play modern, almost avant-garde music in the middle of the night that I didn't get to hear any other time.

Pogo and I were in great spirits. When I pointed out that a particular song being played was special, she seemed to lean in to the radio to hear more clearly. The road was wet and I drove with a little more care than on dry pavement, but the moderating influence of the ocean had kept the ice away.

After Clarke's Beach, the road climbs up through South River and then takes a turn inland away from the ocean. After an intersection at the top of the hill, the pavement takes a steep downturn with a sharp bend at the bottom.

As I approached the bottom of the hill, I could feel the truck drifting across the road. I wasn't going fast, but it didn't respond as I tried to pull back into the proper lane. Time slows down when life spins out of control. It seemed as though I had ages to think and act as the truck neared the shoulder on the left side. I thought it was interesting how the environment this short distance from the sea was different enough that there was black ice on the road. I also thought that this wasn't too bad, and once I hit the gravel on the far shoulder it would be easy to bring the truck around.

My perception of time changed again as the truck hit the gravel. There seemed to be no time from when the front wheels touched the edge of the road to the sudden realization that I was upside down suspended in my seatbelt. My head wasn't in contact with the roof of the truck and I wasn't touching the seat. I put a hand on the roof to support myself and carefully undid the seatbelt. There was the strange sensation of gravity moving me up through the cab of the truck. With a little squirming I crawled out through the gaping hole where the driver's side window had been.

I stood by the side of the truck and assessed the situation. A ditch nearly six feet deep ran by the side of the road, and the truck had rolled over and come to rest face-first in the ditch. The sudden stop of the vehicle had caused all of the equipment in the back to fly forward through the truck. A large, heavy plywood case containing my heftiest gear had been propelled through the front windshield and was lying in the ditch in front of the truck. Every window was broken out. This truck was finished, and I was very lucky.

Pogo poked me with her nose. It was a relief to see her safe and in good spirits. She looked thrilled, in fact, as if she'd come to ask if we could do that again.

But there was work to be done. I crawled back into the truck to dig out my calving equipment. My surgical gear had found its way into the front seat and my calving chains and jack were still in the back.

Obe's barn was only about two miles away, but this was going to be a long trek with all my equipment. As I stepped out on the road, I realized why the truck had left the pavement. The road was so slippery I could hardly stand. It wasn't safe to even walk on this surface.

The shoulder was a little better, so Pogo and I set off on foot for the farm. We hadn't gone fifty yards from the scene of the accident when a truck crawled up beside us. His speed indicated he had either more sense or more experience on these roads than I. When the window rolled down I recognized Donald, a neighbour from my own small village. He worked delivering potato chips to small convenience stores around the Avalon Peninsula and clearly started work early.

I explained my situation, and soon Pogo and I were dropped off at Obe's house by the chip delivery truck.

Obe was standing in the lane between his house and the barn. "Took you long enough."

At the best of times Obe was a difficult man to talk to. His eyes didn't exactly line up. One looked at you and the other pointed up and over to the outside of his head. In conversation with Obe, it was hard to know where to look. Usually we look into someone's eyes to let them know we are intensely interested in what they are saying, or we look away if we are uncomfortable or shy. With Obe, his strange combination of eye directions called out for you to look at his face. But then you had to decide which of his eyes to look at. The straight eye suggested that he was listening to you, but the wild eye suggested his mind was miles away.

After my ordeal, I wasn't in much mood to be chastised for the amount of time it had taken me to get to Obe's farm.

"Look, Obe, I've just totalled my truck. We'll get to your cow, but I'd like to phone my wife first and tell her I'm okay."

"I got no phone."

"How did you call me?"

"Brother Bill next door has a phone. He's up, you could call from there."

Brother Bill lived just a hundred yards away, and judging from the lights and the music, someone was most definitely up. I walked over to Bill's to use the phone. Pogo stayed with Obe, and I imagine they discussed the cow and the accident.

"Mmm hello?" I had clearly woken Ingrid from a deep sleep.

"Hi, it's me."

"What time is it? Where are you?"

"I'm just calling to let you know my truck went off the road and I'm going to need a ride home."

"Are you ready to come home now?"

"No, I just got here. I still have to deliver this calf."

"Okay, give me a call when you're done and I'll come and get you. I'm going back to sleep now."

As I walked back to Obe's, I wondered why Ingrid sounded so unconcerned when I had just been in a potentially fatal accident. Putting that thought aside, I picked up my calving equipment and headed for the barn.

It seemed that in my absence Pogo had completely won over Obe. The gruff farmer was sitting on a bale of hay rubbing the dog's ears as I came in through the door, but he stopped the moment he saw me and said, "Get away, dog."

Over in the corner of the barn, a large white cow was lying on her side and pushing. Her eyes bulged from their sockets as every urge brought a pathetic moan. She was drenched in sweat, and frothy saliva dripped from the corners of her mouth.

Obe had a bucket of warm water ready and a couple of towels. I rolled up my sleeves, washed my arms and reached inside to see where the calf was. It didn't take long to find the cause of the cow's problems.

The calf was coming backwards, with its hind legs oriented forward, and he or she was big.

Sometimes calves do come out backwards. The advantage of trying to deliver a calf in this direction is that only the two hind legs need to be directed out, whereas in a normal delivery, the front legs and the head lead. The disadvantage is that backward deliveries must be done quickly. When a calf is still inside the mother, it gets its oxygen from the mother's blood through the umbilical cord. When calves come out back legs first, the umbilical cord is pinched off once the hind legs are out. As soon as the cord is obstructed, the calf will get no oxygen until its head is in the air and it can take a breath. This means that there must be no delay between the back legs coming out and the conclusion of the delivery.

Feeling the size of this calf, I was concerned that it could end up getting stuck inside and suffocating.

The first order of business was to move the calf so that its hind legs would emerge first. As it was, the calf's rump was jammed into the opening of the mother's pelvis. Her pushing was only making things worse.

I washed up again and placed the palm of my hand against the calf's rear end. Each time the cow would relax after a contraction, I tried to push the calf farther back into the uterus so I could manoeuvre the legs into the birth canal. The problem with this approach was that every time I pushed against the calf, the cow was stimulated to push back even harder. Before long I was drenched in sweat and getting tired. The trick here was to shove hard just as the cow relaxed, to move the calf before she could push back.

After fifteen or twenty minutes with no success, one of my efforts moved the calf back down into the uterus. The calf was now deeper into the cow's abdomen and away from the pelvic opening, easing the pressure on the mother's cervix. She seemed relieved.

Now that the calf was in a better position to work on, I had to pull the legs around so that the hind hooves would lead the way out. I reached in again, found the calf and placed my hand around a hind leg high up in the groin. Feeling my way down the leg, I soon got to the point that I could reach no farther. The calf's hooves were too far away for me to reach. I hooked my fingers into the curve of the hock—the large joint halfway down the leg—and pulled hard. This manoeuvre twisted the legs back at the hips. The bend in the hock meant that the hooves were still facing in the wrong direction, but at least now I could reach them. I repeated this move on the other leg so that I had both legs bent toward me from the calf's hips.

Now I needed to flip around the lower sections of the hind legs so that the hooves faced me. To accomplish this, I put a chain around each hind leg at a level just above the hooves. Once the chains were firmly in place, I pulled them back from outside the cow as I pushed forward on the calf's bottom. With a satisfying pop the two legs straightened out to face me.

Now the calf had to come out. I already had chains attached above the hooves, so it only took a tug to bring the legs up through the pelvic opening and out into the air.

Because I knew the calf was very large and coming backwards, I wasn't going to take any chances with a slow delivery. The calf jack would ensure that the calf would come out as quickly as possible. After lubricating the inside of the cow's birth passage with soap lather, I placed the curved frame of the jack against her back end. I slid the jack along the central tube until it reached the chains attached to the calf's legs.

Jacking a calf out of a cow requires a certain amount of restraint. The jack is capable of pulling with a force of about two thousand pounds, enough to do severe damage to both cow and calf. It is imperative to know whether the calf is small enough to fit through the cow's birth passage without damage. If the calf is too big, a Caesarean section is required.

Luckily, this delivery went smoothly. With a few cranks on the jack, the calf's hips were out and very soon afterwards the whole calf fell to the ground. The newborn bull relieved us all by gasping and blinking his eyes as soon as he was out. Obe and I dragged him up to his mother's head and she began frantically licking the calf and calling out with a pleading moo. I dabbed a little iodine on the navel to prevent infection, and my work was done.

With my gear put away and a bill prepared for Obe, I headed back to Bill's to arrange my ride home.

"Hello . . . ?"

"Hi, I'm all done here. Can you come up and get me?"

"Can't you back your truck out of the ditch?"

"The truck is toast. It's upside down with all the windows broken out."

"What! Why didn't you tell me? Are you okay? I'm on my way." Click.

Perhaps my earlier description of the night's events hadn't contained enough detail. As I waited for my ride home, I thought about the night's adventure. The truck was ruined, but it was only a replaceable machine. Pogo and I were fine, and Obe had a healthy cow and a new calf in his herd.

13. No Bull

THE BULK OF MY WORK didn't feature the drama of surgeries or deliveries. Perhaps the most routine of all large-animal surgeries is a bull castration. Indeed, every spring, just as calvings and associated problems bring the year to a hectic peak, a veterinarian is deluged with calls for bulls to be pinched, cut, nipped, doctored or done.

By the summer of my second year in practice in Newfoundland, confidence was little problem. A few spectacular cures had convinced most of the area's farmers that I might know more than the local experts, and general success had buoyed my own feeling of competence.

When I started work with the government, I was supplied with a dozen pairs of coveralls. These fit fine at first, but with each successive washing they began a race for my knees. By the time the coveralls had seen two years, I looked ready for the floods. Robert, the tall high school student who had performed so admirably in the North River delivery, gave the impression that only major rivers could dampen his cuffs when he wore a pair.

We were having a wonderful day. Calls started with a bunch of bull calf castrations and then a colt with a nasty cut along its side. This was a quick job, a simple matter of cutting away some hair, cleaning the wound and stitching things up. Robert's obvious delight at holding the colt and tying up the final stitches brightened everyone's mood.

Our next call was to a pig that wasn't eating. From a veterinary point of view, Newfoundland's pig population was intriguing. In the 1960s the provincial government had decided to provide the province with a clean slate of pigs. All the pigs resident at that time were removed and replaced.

The new pigs were all SPF, or specific-pathogen-free. They were of the same breeds as before, but special because they had been delivered by Caesarean section from sows raised in carefully isolated facilities. As a result, they were free from a number of the most common swine diseases. This meant I didn't see many of the diseases I had learned about in school. When I saw a sick pig, the number of possibilities was automatically narrowed down far beyond what would be seen in other parts of the country.

We arrived at a small house that looked like it could have used a new coat of paint a few years back. The woman of the house took us out to the back where her sow was housed in a ramshackle barn. I could immediately see that the pig was quite sick. She lay on her side, uninterested in our entrance into her domain. A quick look at her revealed raised red areas along her belly and side. The distinctive diamond shape of the lesions left no doubt of the cause.

Erysipelas is a bacterial disease that is often passed from wild birds to pigs. I looked around. Sure enough, the open spaces in the sides of the barn made it easy for birds to come in to share the pig's feed.

It was always a pleasure to come across problems that were as simple to diagnose as this pig's. Robert was delighted to inject a shot of penicillin into the muscle in the side of the pig's neck. We reassured the owner that the pig would be up and around in no time and we left pleased with how well the day's cases were going.

I usually listened to the radio when on the road between calls, but with a keen student in the truck, it was fun to talk of interesting cases and rehash the morning's work. We were discussing different ways to hold down animals for sutures when we arrived at Mrs. Spracklin's. Both of us were eager and ready to unman her bull.

As we pulled into her drive, Mrs. Spracklin came out of a small shed drying her hands on an old piece of towel. She was a heavy-set, no-nonsense woman dressed in a well-worn set of coveralls. It was pretty clear that it was she who did most of the work with the animals on the family farm.

Her first words as we left the truck were, "Aren't you boys a little young to be at this?" The woman had a lot of nerve. Despite our high-flying pant cuffs, I thought we looked the picture of professional competence. I was absolutely certain that the two of us could handle a bull castration. There was no point in letting her poor observational powers get us upset.

With great seriousness, I explained that I had just finished high school and was doing this for a summer job. When she mentioned the procedure at hand, I let slip that I had never done one before. The look of horror on her face made me confess the truth that I was quite qualified and in fact had castrated eight bulls just that morning.

Two bovine heads peered across a fence at us. I dropped a loop of rope over the head of the closest one. I nimbly vaulted the fence and in short order had fashioned a halter and secured the animal to a fence post. Certainly, I thought to myself, this display of animal restraint will have her eating her words. Too young, indeed!

"We'll have this one done in a minute," I called over.

The woman and her recently arrived daughter burst into laughter. "You won't be doin' that one."

I looked down between the back legs—and noted an udder where I was expecting to find testicles. Turning my head to hide the rosy hue no doubt coming to my face, I removed the halter from the young female. The rope went efficiently onto the bull and the castration was done smartly.

At the conclusion of the procedure, both the bull and the vet had a little less swagger.

14. The Cat in the Trap

MY PRACTICE WASN'T ALL about cows, horses and pigs. There were also moose, otters and lynx to be looked after. Many of my opportunities to work with wild animals like these came from my association with Salmonier Nature Park. In the 1970s the park was opened as an educational centre to display the indigenous wildlife of the province. Wild birds and mammals were brought in and housed in large areas similar to their natural environment. As the park developed, the staff acquired expertise in handling wild animals both on site and around the province. As well as looking after the health of resident animals, I was often asked to assist when park officials were called out for local wildlife problems.

In one such case, farmers in the nearby village of Colinet were losing sheep to a predator at an alarming rate. Park staff came to the conclusion that the culprit was a lynx. Carnivores kill in characteristic ways, and lynx tend to leave bite marks around the base of their victim's skull.

Lynx are not particularly social animals, and individuals or females with a litter of kittens often live by themselves. The curious aspect of the case of the Colinet kills was that a large number of lambs were being preyed on in a very small area, far more than the average lynx tends to eat.

The park staff concluded that the lynx responsible must be unusually aggressive. When one Colinet farmer reported the loss of over a dozen lambs within ten days, it was clear that something had to be done. Staff set a number of baited traps in the area and checked them several times each day.

One morning, I was visiting the park when the Colinet farmer called in to say that a lynx was caught in a trap on his pasture. Rod and Felix, two experienced animal handlers, planned to put the lynx into a cage and release it in a new location far from any sheep farms. I grabbed my drug box from the truck and the three of us headed out to the pasture in a park pickup.

Lynx have an odd way of reacting to being caught in traps. Many trapped animals will thrash around and injure themselves, but lynx tend to sit quietly.

We all climbed out of the truck and carried a wire-sided cage up to the spot. Sure enough, the animal was sitting up passively. He watched us approach but made no effort to move away or hide himself.

I'm not sure why lynx react this way, but it may have something to do with the way that cats experience pain. I've always believed that cats, both domestic and wild, feel pain especially keenly. It may be that when lynx are caught in a trap the pain paralyzes them, because they know that movement will only increase the hurt.

I warily circled the lynx to size up his situation. He didn't even turn his head in order to keep an eye on me. The animal was caught in the trap by one foot—a hold tentative enough that a sudden bolt might free him.

We all retreated from the lynx and discussed our approach to moving him. He would need some kind of sedation before we could carefully assess him, and the only practical way to get the drug into him was by injection.

Our options were to toss a dip net over the animal or to needle him unnetted as he sat in the trap. We decided to inject him where he was, with one person holding the dip net ready to cover him if he went into action.

I pulled a 5-cc syringe from my drug kit and drew up a dose of ketamine, a quick-acting and very safe anaesthetic. I stepped around behind the lynx. Again, he paid no attention to me. To check how much he would put up with, I gingerly reached out and touched a finger to his hind leg. I half expected the animal to wheel and attack me, but it made no response at all.

With this reassurance, I pushed the needle quickly into the big muscles of his hip area. Again there was no response. The final test would be what he would do when I injected the drug. I had seen domestic cats object violently when injected with ketamine—it seemed to cause them pain.

But to my surprise, the wild cat didn't react at all. He didn't even lower his head to look at the syringe as I gave him a full dose.

We all sat on the grass waiting for the drug to take its effect. In a few minutes the lynx was teetering from side to side. His eyes opened wide and his head bobbled. Ketamine causes hallucinations, and no doubt the lynx was seeing something even more strange than these people who had stuck a needle into him.

When he was clearly no longer aware of the world around him, I was able to get a closer look at how he was caught. The jaws of the trap had closed around one toe on his left front foot. The trap was so close to the end of his toe that it had crushed the nail and split the skin at the end of the digit. A minor repair was in order.

"Let's get him back to the park as fast as we can and maybe I can stitch him up before he wakes up."

We pushed the cage over the lynx, unfastened the trap from its stake in the ground and placed the cage, lynx and trap into the back of the truck. Everyone jumped in and we made a dash for the park.

It took us only fifteen minutes to get back, and we all realized that time was ticking away on our anaesthesia. I knew it would take all the time we had to fix up the lynx's foot.

The truck flew down the service road to the animal care centre at the park and we jumped out and ran inside with the cage. The room we used for surgery was small but well lit and had a solid stainless steel table to work on. We opened the cage and lifted the lynx and trap onto the table.

As soon as one of the staff sprung the trap, I began to trim hair away from the affected toe. With a closer look and the trap gone, I could see that the damage was only skin deep. Although the toe bone at the end of the lynx's foot was delicate, it had not been broken by the trap.

With a pair of heavy scissors, I snipped off the crushed end of the nail. I opened a pack of absorbable suture with a straight needle attached. There was no way we would be taking these stitches out, so I wanted material that would dissolve.

Seeing the way that the split in the skin ran up the side, I decided that I could close the wound with four stitches, three if we were pressed for time. The first stitch went in quickly, and I tied a speedy surgeon's knot. Rod was used to fast surgery on wild animals and he had a pair of scissors ready to cut off the excess suture. The second stitch was a little harder to place, as it was farther up between the lynx's toes. Before sticking the needle through the skin, I bent the needle so that it would come up between the toes to a place where I'd be able to get at it more easily. There was no reaction to the needle piercing the skin, but the cat flinched when I tightened the knot. Rod cut the extra suture away as soon as the knot was tied.

With the movement of the famously aggressive lynx, I decided that the third stitch would be all we tried. This would close the gap left between the first suture and the end of the toe. Driving the needle through the skin made the animal flinch more than before. Everyone in the room was tense as I clasped the end of the suture in my needle drivers to tie the knot.

With the first tug on the suture the lynx exploded into consciousness. Everyone in the room moved at once. I finished two throws in the knot, dropped the needle drivers, made a quick snip and grabbed the lynx by the back of the neck. Felix closed the door to the surgical room and Rod lifted the cage to the height of the table.

I quickly slid the lynx across the stainless steel table and into the cage. Rod slammed the cage door shut and snapped the latches.

The three of us exhaled a deep breath. It took us a few seconds to compose ourselves enough to talk.

"That was great fun."

"Yeah, nothin' to it."

15. Special Delivery

EVERY YEAR, in the early spring, most of my attention was captured by the needs of the animals that were delivering the next generation. Deliveries of calves, sheep and goats were a routine part of my job, so it is fortunate they were also my favourite part of veterinary practice. They were a little different than most of my other work, as they were not about sickness. Animals on farms normally deliver their young without any assistance from farmers or vets. Nature is allowed to take its course, and most of the time everything works out well.

Only when an expectant mother runs into trouble is the vet called. Even when there is a problem, the animal isn't sick. Usually the fetus is too big or in the wrong position. The vet's challenge is to find a way to get the unborn animal out of its mother without harming either one of them.

One year, there was one special delivery that monopolized the interest and discussion in our house. Ingrid was nearing the end of her first pregnancy. We woke one morning to a gentle snow falling. Out our bedroom windows we could see the calm ocean drinking up flakes. Inside, the tone was not so serene. Ingrid sat up as she came awake.

"You gotta get me to the hospital, now!"

"Okay, let's go."

Ingrid seemed calm and determined as she pulled on her clothes. I couldn't find my socks and for some reason my pant legs twisted in a way that made pulling them on more complex than I ever remembered. By the time I was dressed, Ingrid had wolfed down a bagel and was waiting at the door with her winter coat on.

"What's holding you up?"

"I'm fine, I'm fine. Don't worry about me. I'll get the car keys. I'll be down in a minute. I've just got to brush my teeth."

It would be a great exaggeration to say that I was calm about the imminent arrival of our first child. I hauled on my coat, ran out the door and started up the truck.

Ingrid waddled over. "What are you doing in the truck?"

"Oh—oh, sorry, it's just my normal routine to get in the truck every morning. I'll get the car."

"Never mind. You've got this going, we might as well take it."

Ingrid hauled herself up into the cab and pulled on her seatbelt. Somewhere in my addled head, a real possibility of slipping off the road had settled in. I drove the short distance to the hospital with as much care as I've ever put into a drive.

By the time we got to the hospital, Ingrid's contractions had settled down. Still, she recognized that the birth was about to happen, and we continued inside. As a physician at the hospital, Ingrid knew the inside of the building well. Today she was to see it from a different perspective.

We checked in, and Ingrid was given a gown and directed to a room where a number of expectant mothers were congregated. She climbed up into a bed, and I ruffled through the pages of an old home decorating magazine. "Why don't you go on to your office," Ingrid suggested. "I'll have them call you if anything happens. You aren't being much help here."

I agreed completely with her assessment of my usefulness and was happy to get away from the intense pressure of nothing happening.

The sandy brick building that housed my office still wasn't open when I pulled the truck up to the staff entrance. To keep occupied, I unlocked all the doors and started turning lights on around the office. With this out of the way, I went down to my lab and began straightening out the drugs in the pharmacy section.

Half an hour after I arrived, opening time came around, and the government agriculture employees who worked in the office began to trickle in. Sharon took off her coat, tossed a brightly coloured scarf over a chair and sat down at her desk.

"What ya up to today, sweetie?" she asked as I directionlessly wandered by.

"Ingrid's in the hospital waiting to deliver."

"What are you doing *here*?"

"Ah, there's nothing for me to do there. They'll call me if anything happens."

"You're crazy. You should be at the hospital."

"I'm heading back down to the lab to clean things up a bit."

"You're crazy."

I had just returned to the pharmacy when I heard the phone ring. Sharon beat me to answering. After a moment, she called, "Andrew, come up here!"

I ran up the hall and sat like an expectant pup in front of her desk. "What is it?"

"That's Craig on the phone. He's got a goat having some trouble with delivering kids. Do you want me to pass this along to the vets in town?" The practice in St. John's covered my area when I was away or sick. It seemed to me that as I wasn't sick or away I should answer the call. "Here, hand me the phone."

"Hey, Doc, how is ya? Me goats is 'avin' some trouble getting the young ones out this morning."

"Okay, Craig, I'll be right up."

"You're crazy," Sharon declared for the third time. "Say hi to Ingrid for me when you do see her."

I have to admit that I was relieved to get this call. I really was going crazy, waiting for information about my wife and her labour. Complications are rare when children are born, but I'd seen nothing but complications in the deliveries I'd been involved with as a vet. Given my experience, I was bound to be a little worried.

Outside, the snow had started coming down harder and the wind had picked up. As luck would have it, Craig's place was just around the corner from the hospital. He was one of the few farmers that still kept animals in the relatively suburban setting of Carbonear. When you drove by his neat bungalow, there was no hint that the back yard had a small barn with a half-dozen goats in residence.

"Whaddaya at this fine mornin', Doc?" Craig was from Upper Island Cove and he retained a sharp accent that set him apart from his neighbours in Carbonear. He had a sporty air to him. Though well past forty, he was always dressed in clothes that would more befit a teenager. His outfit was customarily set off by a brilliant white pair of running shoes with the laces left untied.

"Big day for me, Craig. My wife's expecting. Likely our baby will be born today."

"Right on, skipper. Let's have a look at my kids first."

Craig's barn was always neat. There was never manure or dirt on the floor to take the shine off his shimmering running shoes. He was also well prepared for my visit. A bucket of steaming water, a bar of soap and a neatly folded towel were set on a stool outside one goat pen.

"Come on out here now, my love."

Craig reached in and pulled a distended and upset goat from her quarters. She bawled as I cleaned her back end and gently reached in to assess her progress. I could feel three front legs trying to come out. It was a simple job to find the two that belonged together and push the third back out of the way. With this done, a tug on the remaining two legs brought out the first kid. He sputtered and shook his head as he hit the air. It was a beautiful black-and-white male.

Calvin was quick with the towel and had the kid clean and up to its mother's face by the time I reached in again. The second kid came even easier, a sister for the first.

I cleaned up quickly and wrote Calvin a bill. When he offered a cup of tea, I declined, thinking I should check in with my wife.

At the hospital, I parked the truck in the spot reserved for Ingrid in the doctors' parking lot and rushed in the door. On the obstetrical floor, the spotless nurse smiled and directed me into the room that Ingrid was still resting in.

"How's it going?"

"I'm glad you're here. I think I'm about ready to go." Ingrid spoke through clenched teeth. It seemed to me that she was very ready. A nurse passing by saw her and insisted that she move into the delivery room straight away.

The same nurse directed me to a change room where I got into a scrub suit and a cloth cap. This was likely a good idea. Although I had washed up after the vet call and taken off my coveralls, there was still a definite reek of goat to my clothes. By the time I reached the delivery room, Ingrid was up on a table and having hard contractions. The room was a lot cleaner than what I was used to for delivery.

"I delivered two kids this morning," I said, trying to inject a little levity into the situation. "Your turn, and you only have to deliver one."

From Ingrid's reaction I decided that it might be best to be quiet for a while.

A second nurse came into the room. "They called the obstetrician, but he's having some trouble getting out with all of this snow."

Ingrid clenched her face from a deep contraction and panted, "I don't think I can wait for him."

The nurses looked at each other with concern. "Who's going to do the episiotomy?"

"I could do that," I said. "I've done loads of them."

The two nurses looked at me in horror. "Forget that. We'll wait for the obstetrician."

Perhaps, I thought, I should stay quiet. None of my suggestions that morning were going over well.

The obstetrician did arrive within five minutes, and shortly afterwards, Ingrid delivered a beautiful eight-pound baby boy. One of the nurses cleaned him up, and after Ingrid's turn, I held him in my arms. As I looked down into his eyes, I marvelled at this new person, our son Liam.

My work with animals was put into sudden, sharp perspective. It was important—but nothing could touch the feelings and life-changing impact of the delivery of our little boy.

16. The Cruel Sea

THE GREAT LOBSTER HUNT had a 3 a.m. start. An anaesthetist friend, Paul, and I had been invited to play fishermen
by a farmer who went out for lobster each morning. Working
around the fishing communities of coastal Newfoundland,
and admiring what looked like a wonderful way of life, I
often wished that I could try at least a day out on the water.
Richard the farmer went out early, though, and lived two
hours away, so the adventure began with bleary eyes and
uncertain stomachs.

We stumbled into the truck and set off. Though long, the
drive to the Cape Shore region of the Avalon Peninsula is
always breathtaking, and a chill in the air and the rising sun
brings everything into sharper focus. The beauty of the Cape
Shore is severe; the wind blows hard and the rocks are
exposed. Trees that manage to survive have only stunted
limbs on the side of the prevailing wind. They always seemed
to be begging for some painter or photographer to come
along to take at least their image to a more sheltered place.

The early-morning scenery and chill had us ready for the
ocean. In Richard's house in Angels Cove, the wood stove
was crackling and breakfast was waiting. We'd had a bit to
eat before we set out, but our two-hour drive had us ready for

a second filling. Over bacon, eggs, toast and orange juice, our congenial host asked us whether we had taken any Gravol. The thought of seasickness had not had the chance to enter either of our minds this early in the day. Besides, there was a matter of pride here. Neither Paul nor I had spent much time on the water, but we didn't want to begin the day with an admission of weakness.

"There was a guy just down the road from here," Richard began, "who got sick every morning he went out fishing." There was an extended pause while no one spoke. "And he fished full-time for eighteen years. Once he threw up, he was fine for the day, but every single day he was on the water, he got sick."

There was another pause as Richard, Paul and I shot glances back and forth.

"If you'd like a Gravol," Richard said to no one in particular, "there's lots in the bathroom."

One possibly tall story wasn't going to scare real men into a pharmacological retreat from the realities of the sea. We boldly shook our heads.

"The last time I took a couple of young fellers out fishing they got pretty sick." Another pause. "And it wasn't nearly as rough as it is this morning." It hadn't seemed that rough to us as we drove in, but neither of us could resist peering sidelong out the window in the direction of the ocean.

"We were out about twenty minutes when they started to throw up," Richard continued. "I don't think I ever saw anybody get as sick as those kids. First it was their breakfast coming up and eventually it was nothing but white foam. When we got back to the wharf, the two of them were lying in the bottom of the boat and kind of twitching. I had to grab them by the belts and lift them out of the boat. Funny, they haven't been out since." He gulped down the last of his coffee. "Are you sure you don't want any Gravol?"

Paul smiled at me with hesitation and I looked weakly back. It was obvious to us that this was to be a game of nerves.

"No, thanks," I answered, a little less definitely than before.

"Me neither," added Paul.

Richard sensed our weakening and seized the offensive. "Did you hear about the guy that came down here last year and died?" There was a pause that expected no response. "He was out fishing and started to get sick. By the time they got him in, he was in convulsions. They flew him to Montreal, but he died the next day. Now, a lot of people here say he died from seasickness, but I don't believe that. You can get pretty bad from being seasick, but you can't actually die from it." He looked out toward the ocean. "At least, I don't think you can."

"Okay, I'll have a couple of Gravol."

My partner had deserted at the height of the skirmish, but I was determined to carry on. I glowered at Paul as Richard strutted off to the bathroom. He returned with two Gravols and a glass of water. It appeared that one intimidated land-lubber was enough for him for now. Paul dropped his eyes as he placed the Gravol pills in his mouth and swallowed. Secretly, I envied him. Perhaps I was reading too much into all of this, but it seemed to me that Richard knew that he had beaten us both. Paul had been forced by Richard to eat humble pills, and now I'd been forced by my pride not to eat humble pills. Perhaps Paul had chosen the wiser path.

With breakfast over, it was time to prepare for the sea. While Richard found oilskins and a pair of red-toed rubber boots for Paul, I brought in my fishing finery from the truck. My rain clothes certainly had a well-lived-in appearance from all the post-mortems and rainy-day surgeries they had been through. My dirty baseball cap finished the look.

"You guys look just like real fishermen," Richard commented. "A pair of cuffs each and you'll be all set."

Every fisherman I ever saw wore white cotton gloves if they wore anything on their hands. But there was something wrong with these. They were just too white; they were brand new. Set off against our filthy raincoats, boots and hats, they seemed to glow. I felt like Mickey Mouse.

The three of us piled into Richard's old pickup. It took a couple of coughs, but the truck did start and we lurched off for the wharf, five miles down the highway in St. Bride's.

"Buddy up the road here parked his truck on the hill beside the wharf," Richard told us. "I guess his brakes weren't that good because when he got back from fishing the truck was in the water. They managed to haul it out, but it never was much good after that. My brakes aren't too good either."

During the long pause that followed, Paul and I wondered if Richard's truck might be a candidate for an unscheduled dip in the sea. That would be especially bad if it happened before we got the chance to jump out.

"I don't park up on the hill anymore."

We silently sighed with relief in the knowledge that we would be safe—for at least the parking portion of our fishing trip.

It was still cold and early as we walked from the truck to the edge of the water. St. Bride's has a well-protected deep harbour. An artificial breakwater stretches out from the shore and across, to keep the anchored fishing boats isolated from much of the force of the Atlantic. Richard's boat was moored out about fifty yards into the harbour, with a small punt nestled in beside it. From where we stood, two ropes ran out to the smaller boat, and with an ingenious pulley system, Richard began to pull the punt in to where we waited on the shore.

As the punt came closer, I realized that this was a rather tiny vessel. With Paul in the bow, myself in the stern and Richard between us on the oars, there would be no room for more passengers.

"It's very deep here," Richard began once we were out about ten yards. "You wouldn't believe it, but it's twenty faddom. A few years back a couple of guys got on the beer and decided to go out to their boat on a rough night after dark. They never did find them."

Somehow, this didn't surprise me. There was a definite tone to the stories we had been told so far. The width of our tiny punt made it quite easy to believe that even without being on the beer it would be quite possible to end up in the drink.

We arrived at Richard's boat without incident. She was about twenty feet long, with a small windowless covered wheelhouse. The boat's motor started without hesitation and ran smoothly. The contrast with the truck's condition said much about the priorities of a fisherman.

As we steered among the other boats in the harbour, I

stood on the deck feeling smug. With my lived-in rainsuit and a confident stance, I felt that I fit right in. But I soon noticed that every fisherman on board every boat we passed stopped to stare at the two outsiders on the water. No doubt they knew everyone who used the harbour and were wondering who these newcomers were, and not just admiring our near-fluorescent gloves.

The day was calm and the four-mile run down to Richard's traps passed without incident. The buoys marking his traps were within sight of his house, and it struck me as odd that we'd had to drive and then sail so far to get within a few hundred yards of where we had set off from. Richard had about forty traps set out, and each day of lobster season began with his checking all of them. We approached each buoy, leaned over the gunwales, took hold of the line and pulled the traps up from the bottom. It was exhilarating work, hard on the back and rough on the hands. Even with our gloves it was easy to see why fishermen develop the pink swollen hands they always have. On a calm day it was hard work; I wouldn't want to try it with the water rough. After hauling eight traps into the boat and rebaiting those whose fatal attractions were gone, we finally got a lobster. Richard undid the door on the top of the trap and spilled the unfortunate crustacean out on the deck.

"Grab that fella now, lads."

The lobster turned his alien eye stalks toward us and swung his arms back and forth while snapping his claws. I'm not sure what kind of things lobsters think about, but this one was definitely daring any of us humans to make a move toward him.

Paul and I looked at each other and said nothing. We had developed some sort of ESP that made it unnecessary for either of us to say "Are you nuts?" or something along those lines. We understood each other completely, and neither of us made a move.

"I'm just kidding you, guys." Richard reached into a wooden box for a strange-looking pair of pliers. He bent down, held the lobster by the back, and using his pliers, placed an elastic band around each claw. Paul and I were convinced that this operation was made easier because we were distracting the miniature monster.

It wasn't a great day for lobsters; we got only six from all the traps that we pulled. It was great exercise pulling the traps up out of the water, and eventually both Paul and I managed to catch a lobster from the bottom of the boat and apply the elastics.

"The tide's not right today," Richard advised us. "There's no sense in pulling the rest of the traps today. We'll go have a look at the net."

As he turned to put his motor in gear, a loud whooshing came from the side of the boat just as a shiny piece of black skin eased forward through the surface of the water. A minke whale had come up for a breath of air within twenty feet of us. Minkes are amongst the smallest whales found in the North Atlantic, but at up to thirty feet in length they are still quite impressive. Perhaps *impressive* isn't an appropriate word for the feeling one of these inspires when they surprise you next to a small boat out in the ocean.

The whale made one more pass before he tired of our little

sideshow and headed off for bluer pastures. Richard told us that while it was common for the whales to come around boats while people were fishing, it was extremely rare for them to hit the boats. It doesn't seem too surprising to imagine that the whales should know what they are doing and where they are going in their own element. It shouldn't be any more likely for a whale to hit a boat than for a moose to run into a tree in the woods

Richard turned the boat back toward St. Bride's and his nets. After a short run we came upon two buoys bouncing up and down in the ocean. Richard produced a five-foot pole with a hook on the end and instructed us to grab one of the buoys as he passed by. We amazed ourselves by catching it on the second pass. Catching this bobbing bit of plastic looked simple until I stood there eying the buoy as it bounced up and down to a different rhythm than my attempts to stay upright and inside the rocking boat.

Paul and I grabbed the line attached to the buoy and started to pull. Richard had busied himself at the other end of the boat sorting out lobsters and mucking with the engine, and we saw our chance to make ourselves useful. Yet as much as the two of us heaved on the line, we were barely making progress moving the rope out of the water. Our uncanny extrasensory abilities cut in again as Paul and I wondered in unison what could possibly be on the end of that rope. After a few seconds of playing around the edges of that idea, we turned to each other with the sudden realization that Richard usually fished alone. What kind of man was this who could by himself pull up this load that two of us were barely able to budge? These thoughts spurred us on to further exertions and a great amount of grunting that finally brought the net anchor to the side of the boat.

We looked wide-eyed at what broke through the surface: a chunk of concrete the size of a small kitchen table and nearly a foot thick. Our respect for Richard increased as the two of us struggled to tip the monolith into the boat.

Richard had finished his work at the other end of our craft and he took off his hat and scratched his head as he looked at us slumped over this concrete mass that had drained every bit of our strength.

"Lads, usually I use that thing for bringing up the anchor." He jerked his thumb at the electric gurney situated just behind us. "That's great, though, saves wear on the machinery," he said with a great effort to keep his smile from exploding into laughter. "We'll use the gurney to bring in the rest of the net."

He pulled a piece of the net around the wheel of the gurney and flipped a switch. The wheel jerked to life, and as it turned it pulled the net effortlessly into the bottom of the boat. My eyes avoided Paul's and I doubt he looked at me.

Soon we were joined in the boat by a collection of the strangest-looking fish I had ever seen. Growing up in mainland Canada, I was used to the regular fish-like fish that fresh water grows. I never ceased to be amazed by the bizarre creatures that came out of the salt water. Lumpfish, for example, are rotund little beings that look pretty much the same from the front and the side. As we pulled them from the net they sat on the deck inflating and deflating. After we had filled the bottom of the boat and pulled in the second anchor (much more easily than the first), Richard picked up one of the fish.

The lumpfish has an appendage like a suction cup on its underside that Richard used to fasten the fish onto the gunwales. I'm sure that isn't what these suckers are designed for, but it certainly worked well. Richard took the cigarette from his mouth and stuck it into the fish's mouth. With his puffing, the fish quickly drew down the ash from the cigarette, and soon smoke was coming out his gills.

"I just had to show you that, lads, but you know I don't really think it's fair to the poor fish. We'll let this fella go." He returned the fish to the smoke-free security of the sea.

"Now, we've got to put this net back in the water. We'll drop this anchor back overboard and I'll back up the boat until the net is set. Soon as the whole net's in and she's tight, we'll throw the second anchor in as well. I must warn you, lads, to keep your feet up out of the way of the net as she's playin' out. She moves off shockin' fast and it would be easy to get your feet caught in there. A few years back a feller from Placentia was setting out his net when his buddy got his feet tangled up. The skipper didn't notice the other feller gone until the whole net was put out. Drowned him."

Being pulled to the bottom of the ocean tied to a giant concrete anchor didn't sound like a great idea. Paul and I climbed as high up the gunwales as possible for the setting of the net.

The net was set without incident and we stopped to relax and have a smoke. Well, Richard had a smoke; Paul and I just sat and enjoyed the scenery. The thrill of first setting out in the boat and the excitement with the lobsters, the whale and the blowfish had so preoccupied me to this point that I had not given a thought to seasickness. Now, sitting relaxed without distraction, I started to notice how uncomfortable the rising and falling of the boat was making me. The more I thought about this feeling, the worse it became. Before long, I was deep into the kind of seasickness that makes you believe a quick death would be a mercy. Perhaps I should have kept my feet down in the bottom of the boat while that net whizzed by toward the peace of the ocean floor.

Work for the day was over, though, our lovely little harbour was within sight, and this miserable condition would soon end. I'm sure I hid my discomfort; there was no need to say anything out there in the quiet of the sea. All I had to do was force a small smile and hope no one noticed the greenish hue to my complexion. Had Richard sensed my state? His reluctance to start for home and then his second and then third cigarette made me wonder.

At long last he threw his third cigarette butt into the water. "It's time to head home, lads." With that, he stood up and walked back to the wheelhouse. Finally. To no one in particular and completely under my breath, I said, "Thank you, thank you, thank you."

Our last stop before home was at a group of wooden boxes floating just inside the shelter of the harbour. Richard pulled us up alongside one of them. He opened the lid to show a teeming mass of lobsters. After some sorting and rejecting of smaller lobsters, he pulled out two of the biggest creatures.

"How many of these do you lads want?" he asked.

Despite our protests, he insisted that we must take some lobster home for a meal. When we finally agreed to take a lobster each, he looked disgusted.

"One lobster, that's not even a snack. Here, take a half-dozen each, that'll fill you up good."

We finally wore him down to giving us four lobsters each. For a day's fishing that yielded only six lobsters, I felt we were well compensated. We really hadn't been much help—in truth we were probably more in the way. But perhaps we had entertained Richard as much as he had entertained us.

17. Impress a Student

VETERINARY MEDICINE has always been a very difficult profession to enter. In any elementary school, you'll find more children who want to be vets than want to be doctors to humans. But for every ten positions for medical students in Canada, there's just one veterinary space.

The local high school students who accompanied me for work experience ranged from the brilliant to the mediocre. A number of them went on to careers in the profession, but some never had a chance. I always liked to encourage students, but at times it was difficult. Very high marks were required to even get an interview.

Sometimes I could tell within the first few minutes in the truck when a student just wasn't cut out for vet work. One fellow produced a pack of cigarettes as soon as he settled in the passenger seat. I quickly let him know that no one smoked in my truck. He huffed, looked disgusted and turned his head to the side window for the rest of the trip. When we stopped to look at a horse, he stomped over to a corner of the field to smoke and never saw any of the procedure. So at noon, even though I had a full afternoon booked, I told him there wasn't anything else coming up that would interest him.

When students were keen and engaged, I always hoped

their time with me would heighten their interest in becoming a vet. But it didn't always work out that way.

David was a clever and enthusiastic student who lived near the biggest farm in the practice, one I visited every two weeks for a routine checkup on the herd. When I drove up to Dave's house in Mackinsons, he was sitting on a rock in his front yard. On the ground beside him were a pair of boots and a bagged lunch. During the short drive to the farm he asked questions about what we would be seeing and doing that day.

As well as a herd-health visit to the dairy barn and a check on some pigs, a sick cow needed attention at the farm. The pigs were first. Dave and I walked through all of the pig barns to check that the animals were happy and healthy. There were no major problems, and we spent some time talking about whether some of the young pigs were a little overcrowded in their pens.

We washed up and changed into clean coveralls for our visit to the dairy. Wal and Tom, the herdsmen, were cleaning the alley between the rows of cows as we came in. Tom continued on with his work while Wal came into the office to look over the past week's records. Everything was going well, he said, except that one cow hadn't been eating for a couple of days.

Before we got to the sick cow, we would check on the reproductive status of the herd. Dairy farming is all about making milk. Cows produce milk when they have calves. The goal with individual cows is for them to have a calf and then produce milk for about three hundred days. The cow then gets a break for about sixty days before she is expected to have another calf. This works out to a cycle of about one full year: a cow's pregnancy lasts around nine months, leaving her with three months to get pregnant after a delivery. Breeding can start at around two months after giving birth, and it isn't the romantic affair one might imagine—no bulls are directly involved. Frozen semen, stored in liquid nitrogen, is introduced by the farmer into the cow's reproductive tract through a straw. If the procedure is done at just the right time, the cow's eggs will be fertilized and a new life will begin. The cow must be bred efficiently for the whole cycle to stay on track. In order to have a constant supply of milk, dairy farms want cows calving throughout the year. If all the animals in a farm had the sixty-day dry period at the same time, there would be no milk for about two months.

To keep up with this demanding schedule, dairy farmers regularly check to see whether cows are pregnant. A veterinarian without any special equipment can diagnose pregnancy as early as thirty days after breeding. If a cow turns out not to be pregnant, it's critical that the farmer makes sure she will be soon.

I pulled on my shoulder-length glove and lubricated it as Dave and I followed Wal out into the barn. He stopped at each cow that had been bred more than thirty days before, and I performed an examination. It's not an easy procedure. You have to feel the uterus through both the plastic glove and the wall of the rectum. Although the glove kept me clean, it also dulled the level of sensation my fingers could appreciate. In a pregnant cow, the uterus will slip or pop subtly in your fingers as it is gently palpated. When a cow is not pregnant, further palpation of the cow's ovaries is done to check for any problems that might be causing her infertility.

After checking a dozen cows, I asked Wal if Dave could have a feel inside a cow closer to delivery. I'd found this was a procedure that separated out the students who seriously wanted to be vets. The ones who complained about having to put their arm up the back end of a cow likely weren't going on. Those whose eyes lit up when they felt the movement of an unborn calf were real vet material.

Wal picked out a cow and Dave pulled on an examining glove. As Wal held the cow's tail to the side, Dave gently reached inside. The concentrated look on his face gave away his excitement at actually doing some vet work.

"Wow!"

That was all it took for me to know that he had felt the calf—and that a future veterinarian was possibly in the barn with me that day.

With the pregnancy checks finished and recorded, we moved on to the sick cow. She didn't look too bad, but her eyes lacked the shine that healthy animals have, and the pile of hay in front of her suggested she didn't have much appetite.

With my stethoscope I listened to her heart and lungs. No trouble there. Next came the digestive system. While listening over the left side of the cow's abdomen, I tapped at her side with an index finger. As I moved the stethoscope around, I came across a section that resulted in a sound like you would hear tapping on an overinflated beach ball. This tone suggested gas under pressure, and the location of this ping indicated a displaced abomasum.

The arrangement of a cow's four stomachs sometimes allows the fourth one to flip over. The abomasum normally sits around the middle of the bottom of the abdomen. When it gets filled with air, it can rise up along one side of the cow.

This cow had a left displaced abomasum, or in simpler terms, a twisted stomach. With the fourth stomach twisted around, it is difficult or impossible for food to pass through the digestive system. The most effective way to put the wayward abomasum back in place is with surgery.

There are a number of ways to correct this problem surgically. My favourite approach was to first lay the cow on her back. In this position the abomasum normally floats back up into a location near where it should be sitting. Once the stomach is in the right place, it can be surgically secured in position.

Wal and Dave put a halter on the cow and walked her from her milking spot to a clean open area. I gave her a very small dose of tranquilizer to make her less resistant to lying on her back. I shaved her belly area with my electric clippers and injected a freezing drug into the area I would be cutting. Anything I could do before putting her onto her back would decrease the time that she would be in that uncomfortable position.

We looped a rope loosely around her neck and then twice around her abdomen. By pulling on the end of the rope, we persuaded her to lie down. Wal and Tom pushed her onto her right side and tied her back legs and then her front legs together. The men each took the rope from a pair of legs and pulled them to the front and back of the cow. With the cow stretched out, I came in close and put my stethoscope to the abdomen. By tapping as I had done before, I was able to locate her abomasum. It was still in the wrong position, high on the left, so I asked Wal, Tom and Dave to slowly push her up onto her back. As the cow rolled, I could hear the stomach moving up to a more normal position. When she was straight on her back, the cow's abomasum was placed just where it should be.

Wal and Tom took their ropes and tied them to the stalls at either end of the opening we were working in, and I prepared the cow's surgical site.

The surgery started well. With a scalpel I made a six-inch incision just to the left of the midline of the cow's belly. Once the cut was completely through the body wall, I could see the distended abomasum. I opened a small hole into the stomach so the trapped air could escape.

My surgical tools were neatly arranged on a surgical drape wrapped around a hay bale. Just as I reached back for a needle and suture material, I saw one of the cow's back legs jerk forward, and with three more kicks the leg was no longer fastened to the stall. The movement of the first leg loosened the rope on the other leg and suddenly I was working in a war zone.

A kick from a cow can cause serious damage. I was far from interested in finding out how hard this one could kick, but nor could I leave the thrashing cow with an open belly and stomach. My only option was to flatten myself down on the cow's belly. So far her kicks were running along her sides and not coming near the middle. Lying along the cow's abdomen, I quickly sewed the abomasum into place and closed the incision. My concentration was tested by the hooves whistling by both sides of my head.

With the job done, I slid forward out of reach of the loose legs. Wal untied the front legs and let the cow over on her side. In this more comfortable position she stopped kicking. Within minutes she was back on her feet. A quick check with the stethoscope confirmed that the abomasum was back in its proper position.

As Tom walked the cow back to her stanchion, I turned to Dave. "How did you like that?"

"Man, that looked dangerous! Do you have to do things like that all the time?"

"No, I've never had anything quite like that before. Usually it's a pretty safe job."

We washed up the instruments, left instructions for post-operative care of the cow and headed off to the next call.

Lefty Mercer wasn't really a farmer. He had one horse, Princess—was every second mare in Newfoundland called Princess?—which I don't think ever did much more than stand in the barn or wander around the small garden next to the house. It seemed that Princess had found something sharp in the barn and had managed to cut open her upper front leg. A nasty gash about seven inches long ran down the front of the leg just at the level of her chest.

This would require a cleaning and a few stitches. After the excitement of the previous call, I was relieved to be working at the front end of an animal. In cows and horses it's usually the back legs that can cause the most damage. Standing just behind the front leg, I was in quite a safe position.

I trimmed away the hair around the cut and cleaned the exposed tissue with warm water and iodine-based soap.

The first injection of the freezing drug lidocaine went smoothly. As the second needle slid in through the skin on the side of the wound, the horse gave a small jerk. She definitely felt that one, but she relaxed as I emptied the drug into the tissue.

Perhaps I was a little touchy from the other call that morning, but the horse's movement put me on edge. I was relieved to have the most painful part of the procedure over with. Before starting the stitching, I leaned in for one last close look to decide exactly where the sutures would go.

Just as I brought my face in close, Princess kicked up her front leg. In an instant her knee caught me in the chin and lifted me off the ground. I have no memory of the flight to the back of the horse and out the barn door. The landing was rough; I bounced across the snow just outside to a sitting position. I sat for a few seconds as my post-traumatic confusion passed. Tasting blood, I reached up to my mouth to feel how many teeth had been broken. It was a great relief to feel that the only damage seemed to be cuts on the inside of my lips.

As I stood, I noticed Dave shaking his head and backing away from the barn.

Perhaps the worst of the situation was that the work wasn't finished. To prevent a repeat of this fiasco, we tied Princess's halter down to the rail in front of her and Lefty lifted the front leg that wasn't cut.

The rest of the work went without any special excitement. A few stitches closed the wound, and I gave Princess a shot of tetanus toxoid and penicillin.

Dave didn't say too much for the rest of the day, but I noticed him looking at me rather strangely as we went about the remaining calls. I could only imagine that he was wondering how crazy someone would have to be to do this kind of work.

He was a fine student and pleasant to have on calls, but I'm afraid I didn't inspire him to become a large-animal vet. He never called me again.

18. Hit the Road

THE CAPE SHORE PASTURE was getting a new bull.

Early every spring, small-time cattle owners in Newfoundland would bring their animals to the government-subsidized community pastures and leave them for the summer. For a modest fee, the animals were watched and bred. To ensure that the calves produced were of high quality, only good bulls were allowed in. Ordinary male animals had to be castrated before being accepted into the pasture. Because one bull is sufficient to breed about one hundred cattle, it was possible with some effort to introduce very good genetics into the local herd.

Every year, the managers of the more progressive pastures would expend considerable effort to see that a high-quality bull was available to breed their herd. A second bull was usually put in, in case the star performer didn't live up to his billing. At times—such as this particular spring—the federal government provided bulls with superior genetics.

The Cape Shore pasture was the most isolated in my practice. Getting there involved a long drive off the Trans-Canada Highway. It was some of the most scenic road I covered. The road rose and fell along the coastline of Placentia Bay and offered up postcard views of the undulating shore. More than half of the road was unpaved, and flat tires on this trip weren't uncommon.

This year's federal bull was coming in from Ottawa on a cattle transport truck. The driver made regular runs from the mainland to St. John's and he well knew the condition of the road from the main highway to the Cape Shore pasture. He let the pasture operators know that he would bring the bull as far as the turnoff from the Trans-Canada, but he was not taking his truck down that rough gravel road to the pasture.

No one in the area had a cattle transport truck, and the bull was too massive to be carried in a regular pickup.

People on the Cape Shore are innovative. Years of isolation has bred an attitude that something can always be worked out with what is available. In true Cape Shore style, the guys from the pasture found a novel solution. One of the farmers worked part-time drawing gravel, and his dump truck would certainly carry a bull.

When the cattle transport driver arrived at the appointed meeting place, no doubt he was surprised to see a dump truck waiting for him.

Rick, the federal agriculture agent who had made the arrangements, met the two trucks at the highway junction to make sure that the bull arrived in good shape. I really don't know how it was done, but with more inventive thinking, the bull was placed in the box of the dump truck. Rick told me later that, a little worried about the unlikely transport, he had followed the truck partway down the road to the pasture.

Only minutes after Rick turned back for home, the bull

jumped out. Had Rick still been following close behind the truck, a ton of bull would have landed on his car.

My phone rang at eight thirty that evening. It was Cyril from the pasture, and he calmly explained that the bull that had come from Ottawa was now running on and around the road leading to Placentia. He wondered whether I might be interested in having a look. Before leaving, I said goodbye to my family—which now included daughters Adrian and Astrid and our new Australian shepherd, Mats. I paused for a moment to watch the kids and their puppy rolling around on the floor in glee.

It was easy to identify the spot where the bull had escaped. An empty dump truck was pulled up on the side of the road, and behind it a police car with red lights flashing. I was amazed that the bull was alive and running after leaping the considerable distance from a moving dump truck down onto the highway. Since he did survive, he was now a major hazard on the road.

When I went over to the truck, Cyril and an assistant were leaned back in their seats with cups of tea.

"Evenin', guys. Where's your bull?"

"He's just over there." Cyril indicated with a twist of his thumb. "We figured we would wait for you to have a look at him before we got him back in the truck."

They didn't seem too excited by the disaster and weren't in a hurry to start examining the bull.

"Ya want a drink before we start, Doc? We got a couple of beers here and a thermos of tea."

"Thanks, guys. Let's have a look at the bull."

I turned from the truck and walked over to the police cruiser.

"G'night, officer. I see they've called you out to see the bull."

"That's right, and this is as close as I'm getting to that monster. I'll watch the traffic while you go see to the bull."

"Do you get much call to see animals?"

"Listen, the last time I got called for something like this was when there was a horse stuck in a well. He looked like he was jammed in pretty good and they asked if I would shoot him. I got off a shot, but he moved his head in time and the noise scared him so much he jumped right up out of the well. Knocked me over and on the way by nearly killed me. I've had enough of this animal racket."

I fetched a flashlight from my truck and coaxed the farmers out of the dump truck. They had been watching the bull and pointed him out, standing about a hundred yards from the edge of the road. As we approached it, one of the farmers sang a wordless Irish-sounding reel. It was one of those *diddly-di de-dum, de-diddly-dee* songs that all sound the same to me. I often wonder if these are real tunes, variations on a theme, or made up on the spot.

The bull was a massive block of muscle. His coal-black coat made it hard to pick out details in the dark, but we could see he was in excellent condition, with an enormous head and neck. For an animal who had recently hit a gravel road at over fifty miles an hour, he looked quite unconcerned. He faced us as we neared him and didn't seem too worried about our presence. When we got within a dozen yards, I circled to see if I could assess the damage. My circling didn't worry him any more than our approach had. He remained immobile, his body pointed toward the two farmers from the dump truck.

"He's a beauty, Doc. He'll give us some wonderful calves this summer."

From a position behind and a little to the side of the bull, I suddenly ran toward him, yelling and waving my arms. The bull slowly turned his head and eyed me with a bored look.

I had to get him to move. Otherwise, I couldn't tell whether he was hurt.

"Guys, we need to get him walking a bit so I can see if anything has happened to his legs. Any ideas?"

"How about this?" Cyril stepped up directly in front of the bull, dipped his head toward the animal and pawed the ground with his foot. The charade was topped off with a quite convincing imitation of a bull roar. The bull swung his head around from me to the farmer and charged.

The most interesting part of the scene was Cyril laughing as he raced across the boggy ground in his rubber boots. His partner found the situation even more hilarious and fell to the ground in mirthful convulsions. Meanwhile, I had serious work to do, and ignoring the two entertainers, I ran alongside the bull with my flashlight trained on his legs.

I could hear a sickening crunch coming from his back end, and his right leg rolled in an unnatural arc with every step. The looseness of the swing indicated that the bones of his leg were not intact. It seemed to me that he had broken his femur.

The bull ran only about twenty yards before he gave up the chase. His heavy breathing and the drool falling from his mouth suggested great pain. The three of us gathered back together.

"Did you see that?" the assistant managed to get out between guffaws. "Buddy would have killed him if he caught him."

"My son, no bull can run like me."

"I hate to tell you, guys, but your best bet is to slaughter that bull right here. He's broken up badly and he'll never be able to breed for you."

"You sure about that, Doc? He's a lovely bull."

"Sorry, Cyril, but that's my opinion."

"How about if you have a look at him in the morning when there's more light?"

"But we can't leave him here all night. He might get on the road and kill someone."

"That's okay. Me'n Aiden'll stay here for the night and watch him."

If they were willing to put this much effort into being sure about the bull, I felt I should do my share as well. It was an hour's drive home, but that inconvenience paled next to sitting up all night in the middle of nowhere watching a bull from a dump truck. I told them I would be back early the next morning and set off for home.

On the drive home I thought how much easier our lives had become since Ingrid had moved from her work as an anaesthetist into family practice. In her new job there was no longer the risk that she would be called out after hours. For years we had juggled both of us being on call. It was a comfort to know that one of us would be at home with the kids every night.

Next morning, I found Cyril and Aiden slumped in the truck exactly as I had found them the night before. Both had a cup of tea in their hands and they had giant grins on their faces. They seemed to be having a wonderful time.

"Have a good sleep, Doc? The bull hasn't moved all night."

They drained their cups of tea, tipped them over and shook them out through the windows before climbing out. The bull also seemed unchanged from the evening before. There was no evidence that he was in any pain, except that he didn't seem to have eaten anything.

When Cyril stepped into his position from the night before, the bull didn't wait for any further provocation. He lowered his head and took four slow but deliberate steps toward the farmer. This time the daylight allowed me a clearer look at the animal's injuries.

"That's enough, Cyril, leave him alone. I've seen all I need to see."

Cyril and Aiden both looked a little disappointed, but they came over to join me.

"He's a mess," I told Cyril. "Looks to me like his pelvis is smashed up as well. There's no way he can work on your pasture this summer and I'm just about certain he will never get over this."

"Can we take him back to the pasture and see how he does?"

"It would be best to put him down now so he doesn't suffer any longer."

"He looks happy to me. I'd like to give him a chance."

I could see that it was going to be impossible to convince them to slaughter the poor bull right away. He did look reasonably comfortable, I had to admit, and if they took it easy going back to the pasture they could get him home without much discomfort.

"If you really think you need to take him back, here's what I'd suggest. Tie him on carefully in the back of the truck, drive really slowly back home and don't give him any antibiotics. If you do decide to slaughter him and there are no drugs in him, at least you can salvage some meat. Does that sound okay?"

"We'll do that."

"If he looks like he's in pain or losing a lot of weight, don't leave him, okay?"

"We can do that."

I left for home with some misgivings about the conclusion of the affair. There was no question in my mind that the bull had injuries he would eventually succumb to. It seemed to me that moving him to the pasture was only delaying the inevitable. Still, the farmers had the bull's best interest at heart and would watch him carefully.

A week later, I heard from Cyril that the bull hadn't eaten for a couple of days and they reluctantly decided to slaughter him. I was consoled by a call from the butcher a couple of days later. The femur and the pelvis were indeed both broken.

19. Post-Mortem on Long Island

MADONNA CALLED ON A Tuesday afternoon. "Could you come to see Fadder's cow?"

"What's the problem?"

"She's dead."

A dead cow isn't an emergency, so I told Madonna that I would call the next morning to make arrangements for the visit. Early on Wednesday I got instructions from Madonna on how to find the house. Despite my confidence that my four-wheel-drive truck could get anywhere, she kept insisting that her father would take me to the cow.

It was cold, cloudy and windy as I made my way up the isthmus connecting the Avalon Peninsula with the rest of Newfoundland. This narrow strip of land where the waters of the ocean on each side of the island come close together seemed to be always draped in fog. This day was looking even greyer and colder than usual.

The village of North Harbour sits on rock around a harbour off Placentia Bay. Madonna's directions were clear, and I easily found her family's house. A petite pretty girl in her middle teens with an old T-shirt and ripped jeans answered the door. The way she carried the infant on her hip made it plain it was hers and her name couldn't be anything but Madonna.

"Come in and sit down, Fadder'll be back before long. Look out on the bay and see if you can see his boat coming in."

It struck me as odd that her father should be out on the bay when he knew that the vet was coming to see his dead cow. But I shouldn't have been surprised; life ambles along at a leisurely pace in the outports. Being late could never be taken as an indication that an appointment wasn't important. There never seemed to be a great hurry to do anything.

"So how far is it to where your cow is?"

"Fadder can usually get over to the island in about forty minutes."

The island! Long Island lies three or four miles offshore, at the head of Placentia Bay. It was time to do some serious rethinking of my day's plans. I had figured on this call using up a good part of the day with an hour and a half's drive each way and perhaps an hour of work. With any luck I would be finishing up some more calls in the early afternoon. But with at least another two hours of waiting for boats and water travel, it looked like most of the day was gone. I declined her offer of tea and sat in silence for what seemed like hours while Madonna preened for and cooed at her baby. She fairly glowed with pride, and she appeared pleased to have someone from outside the village see her beautiful child. Still, I felt like an intruder sitting with this mother and child in their simple home. Poor fragile Madonna seemingly robbed of her own childhood by this baby that made her so happy. Likely happier, I thought, than many of her rich, bored teenage counterparts in the big cities.

Hearing the hum of another boat that sounded to me just

like the other half-dozen boats that we had heard, Madonna jumped up and ran to the window. "It's Fadder."

We climbed into my truck and made our way down the gravel road to the government wharf. A twenty-five-foot longliner drew up dockside and the captain and mate appeared from inside the wheelhouse. Madonna's father was a wild-eyed man with a few days' growth of white beard and an interesting assortment of teeth. His wife followed him up onto the wharf, her rough hands and weathered face attesting to a life devoted more to work than appearance.

The skipper tied off the boat and paused long enough to twist his head in my direction and grunt "Wait here" before heading off toward town.

"I believe he's gone to the store for some beer," Madonna added helpfully.

The day was already shot as far as more calls went, and a few more minutes waiting for a beer run wasn't going to drastically alter things. Besides, there were fishermen to talk to, boats to ogle and plenty of flat rocks to skip over the water.

Father returned in fifteen minutes with a cardboard box with half a dozen bottles of beer rolling around in the bottom. "This'll help with the trip over," he said. "Let's get going."

Because farm animals often lack the consideration to die in easily accessible places, I kept handy a small tackle box containing the necessities for a post-mortem: a knife, a sharpening stone and steel, some dissecting instruments, a few pairs of disposable rubber gloves and various containers and equipment for collecting samples. The box was easy to carry on trips by snowmobile, horse-drawn sled, boat or even on foot to perform a final bit of scientific analysis on some poor departed beast.

With a pair of rubber boots and the box under my arm, I climbed down over the wharf into the boat. I always prided myself in my ability to get myself gracefully from stationary land into a moving boat or back. In all the times I made this manoeuvre, I never once ended up in the water and I always felt I looked somewhat like an experienced seaman. No doubt the fishermen thought otherwise.

The engine roared to life. Madonna cast off the lines securing us to the wharf and she waved to us as we headed off for Long Island. From the shore, the water had looked almost flat, but once we were out of the shelter of the harbour, I could tell this wasn't going to be a smooth trip.

I had two choices of where to sit. The wheelhouse was cramped, loud and choked with fumes from the engine, but it did have the definite advantage of offering shelter. The deck behind the wheelhouse was about six feet by ten feet and offered a rest from the clamour of the engine. It was cold in the wind, and the deck gave at least the illusion of the possibility of falling over the side into the sea.

I chose the wheelhouse and tried to start up a conversation with my shipmates. The father had the wheel and seemed too busy with his beer bottle for any talk, but Madonna's mother and I chatted.

"Do you spend much time over on the island?" I asked her.

"Every spring we pretty well moves out there until the snow comes. We brings the cow over as soon as there's some grass to eat so she gets a summer on the island."

I didn't pursue the matter of exactly how the cow got over to the island. No doubt they tied her on in the back of this little boat and hoped for the best. Try as I might, I could not imagine any simple way of getting a cow either into or out of this boat. Visions of a panicking bovine deciding that she'd like to get off halfway across the bay ran shivers down my neck.

"Have you ever been to Long Island?" she asked me.

"Yeah, I was here two years ago on a kayak trip. A buddy and I paddled over from Arnold's Cove in one of those boats that are about three feet across and eighteen feet long. We spent about a week exploring around the island."

A disgusted grunt came from the wheel, followed by a muttered "Shit!"

"Don't mind him," the missus told me. "Skipper's been going on all morning about government 'angashores and how fast you'd be getting sick out on the bay. Now he figures there's no way you'll be sick if you've been out here in a little boat like that. There's no way you'd catch me dead in that kind of punt out here."

Another grunt from the skipper. "Yer nuts, my son."

This was the typical reaction to kayaking from anyone who spent their lives on the ocean in larger boats. But kayaks are deceptive craft: in practised hands they are as safe as anything on the water. Historical accounts of long voyages and epic whale hunts across the northern extremes of the globe attest to the kayak's seaworthiness.

Another misconception surrounding the kayak is that anyone who would go out in one of these flimsy vessels must be immune to seasickness. Any kind of motion sickness results from the confusion caused by conflicting signals sent to the brain from your eyes and the balance organs in your inner ear. In a small boat, you become one with your vessel. Every part of your body must be acutely aware of every movement, up, down, sideways or over. On larger boats, it is easier for your eyes to focus on parts of the boat and start the cycle of confusion. It has been my experience that the bigger the boat, the easier it is to get sick.

But now I had inadvertently set up a challenge: my kayaking tale had converted my shipmates from the idea that I was a complete landlubber, and I was not about to disappoint them.

As we got farther out into the bay, the wind and the waves increased to uncomfortable proportions. Our boat was small enough to be tossed erratically by each passing wave. A quick look around the diesel-smoke-filled wheelhouse didn't reveal any life jackets. The stench from the engine wasn't helping my stomach, but I couldn't see a safe place to secure myself out on the deck. It seemed a reasonable compromise to jam my legs against one side of the wheelhouse doorway and my back against the other. In this seemingly nonchalant sitting position, I felt I was doing a pretty fair job of masking my growing nausea.

Soon the boat was slipping over the waves at an angle that seemed to me precariously close to the point where we would be turned upside down. My only consolation was the unconcerned look of my fellow travellers. Boats like this one had been on the ocean for ages, and surely an experienced fisherman like the skipper wouldn't be out if there was any chance of sinking his boat.

Thinking that his plans for humbling the government man with seasickness had been dashed, the skipper decided on another tack.

"Did ya hear about buddy that they caught for stabbin' the other feller?"

"You mean that Russian guy?" I had read in the news of a Russian sailor who had been charged for murder after he had supposedly knifed one of his shipmates while working in Canadian waters.

"Yeah, that's him. It's funny, we could stab you out here, throw you over the side, and no one would ever know."

Two could play at this game. I leaned over to my post-mortem kit, threw open the cover and pulled out my knife with its gleaming foot-and-a-half-long blade. "Look at the size of this knife," I said. "If I was crazy, I could murder you and the woman, throw you overboard and run off to Jamaica with your boat."

The skipper roared with laughter and reached back to slap me on the shoulder. "Yer all right," he said. It was as if I had passed some initiation test. Suddenly the skipper came alive with smiles and stories. I sat enraptured by the tales of how his family had been forced off Long Island in the 1960s by government resettlement. They had taken the family house, floated it on oil drums and towed it across the water to their new home in North Harbour. Like many resettled Newfoundlanders, they never completely gave up on their ancestral home and had returned every summer.

There was one story that I could have done without, though.

"My sister Mary spends the whole summer on the island. She comes across once in the spring and she won't go out on the water until the fall."

"That's right," added his wife. "She really hasn't been much good in a boat since that time we flipped over out here."

Great. So it wasn't just my imagination: there really was a chance this boat would capsize. At over a mile off shore, there wasn't a hope that any of us would make it to land.

Suddenly the waves looked like they were getting worse. The larger ones seemed to put the longliner completely over on its side. Water splashed across the deck and the boat pounded down hard with every passing breaker. I was finding it difficult to maintain the image of an experienced seaman. I battled seasickness and fought off the panic that comes with the certain knowledge that your boat is going to tip at any moment.

After what seemed like hours, we pulled into the lee of Long Island and the waves subsided. There is a point just before actually succumbing to motion sickness where all you can do is wish that you could throw up and get it over with. I was extremely close to this place. The calmness took away any fear that we would all be drowned on this trip, but parts of me were still arguing whether a quiet death at sea might be more enjoyable than feeling as miserable as I did.

Finally, we pulled up to a wharf made of the small tree trunks known as longers that were found on the island. The sides of the wharf were eight feet up from the deck of the boat and the construction looked frail, but I needed little encouragement to scramble up onto the top.

The skipper climbed up behind me, fastened the lines from his boat to the wharf and slapped me hard across the back. "Yer a lovely man," he said.

The sickness faded away as I looked out over the little harbour. Even on a windy, overcast day this was a little piece of heaven. Behind the wharf was a field of grass with one small cabin in the middle. A well-travelled footpath ran parallel to the beach to a second cabin nestled in a grove of poplars. The three of us trundled along in our oil clothes and boots, the sound of rubber rubbing against rubber coming up over the wind. The cabin was covered with freshly painted white siding, and I could see curtains in bright colours through the windows.

Inside, a heavy-set, friendly-looking woman rose from a rocking chair to greet us.

"This is Dr. Peacock. He's a lovely man," said the skipper. "If I'd knowed you wasn't a jerk, I woulda made sure Mary had dinner cooked for you. All we have right now is some bread and peanut butter. Make the man a sandwich, maid."

After a short lunch I suggested that we should really have a look at the cow that everyone seemed to have forgotten about.

We all put our coats and boots back on, and our ragged little army marched back to the wharf.

Mary stiffened and bent down low as soon as her feet touched the deck of the wharf. The skipper took her hand with a tenderness and seriousness that I wouldn't have expected and helped her down into a little dory.

This smaller boat was just big enough to seat the four of us comfortably for the short trip across the harbour. Mary sat squeezed into the bow, her knuckles white from her death grip on the gunwales. The skipper was in the stern, a cigarette dangling from his mouth, standing over his antique one-cylinder Acadia outboard motor. These make-and-break engines, or one-lungers as they're also called, had been the standard source of power on the water for decades but had recently become a bit of a rarity. After three or four pulls, the engine sputtered to life and began its distinctive *putt-putt-putt*. There seemed to be something not quite right with the motor, because the skipper had to keep one finger deep inside the mechanism to keep it running. Every time he removed his hand to flick away an ash, the putting threatened to stop.

Poor Mary leaned woodenly forward as if urging the boat to shore as we crossed the calm hundred yards of the small harbour. I could only wonder how she survived the trip from North Harbour and back each year.

The engine roared as we accelerated onto the beach, and as we touched down, Mary was the first to vault over the sides onto the solid, reassuring sand. We pulled the boat safely up onto the shore and walked the short distance to the cow.

The two-day-old carcass was starting to show its age. When a ruminant dies, the micro-organisms in its digestive system carry on producing gas, so the body quickly bloats. This cow looked like a cross between an animal and a balloon. Perhaps it would have been kinder to warn everyone to stand back when I opened up the carcass, but just this once it was time to put the disgusting parts of pathology to work. On the water, I had been out of my element and been the brunt of everyone else's fun. Now it was my turn.

As I drove my knife into the abdomen, a fine spray erupted from the cow with an unimaginably foul stench. My companions turned as one and with a variety of oaths ran from the scene.

Opening the biggest of the cow's four stomachs, the rumen, I soon found the cause of her demise. It always amazed me how much junk collected on the shores of remote places like Long Island. Now I was amazed at how much of it the cow had swallowed. There were plastic bags by the dozen, there were pieces of hard plastic buckets and there were bits of fishing net. It was hard to imagine how the cow got some of these things into her mouth, let alone swallowed them. So much junk had collected inside her that her digestive tract had become completely blocked.

I called everyone over, showed them a selection of what I had removed from the cow and explained how this had killed her.

"You knowed right away what killed her, didn't ya?"

"Well, I guess," I answered with some modesty as I kicked at the dirt and looked down.

"Yer a lovely man."

All this praise and pleasantry was starting to make me feel a little guilty about my callousness with the knife.

We trooped back into the punt and across the little harbour to the wharf.

Mary, the skipper and his wife all insisted that we have another cup of tea before we set off for the mainland in the bigger boat. As we had tea and another slice of homemade bread, the skipper continued to express his amazement at my ability to tell what had killed his cow. Every time he commented, my feat grew in stature.

"You knowed what killed that cow before you even opened her up, didn't ya?"

"Well, actually . . ."

"Yer some man, my son, yer a lovely man."

After tea we all said our goodbyes to Mary and climbed back into the longliner. The rain started up with more serious intent and the wind blew just a little harder than it had on our trip over. The waves were rougher than before, and the boat lurched in ways I hadn't previously imagined possible.

All the way back the skipper carried on his commentary of my miraculous diagnostic powers. I was sure that before we got home, he would have me knowing what was wrong with his cow before he'd even phoned to tell me she was dead.

I sat contentedly in the wheelhouse and scarcely noticed the wind and the waves.

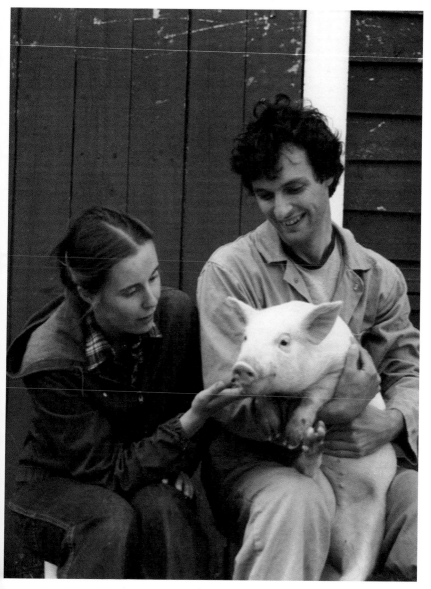
Ingrid and I examine one of my first patients.

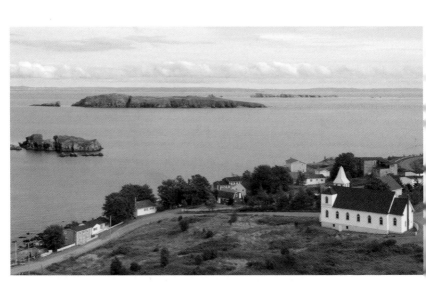

"The sight astonished us": the village of Freshwater, as seen from its rock outcrop.

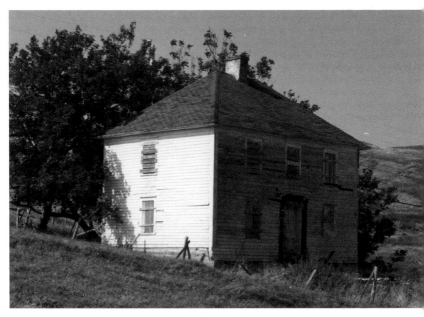

Our perfect house on the ocean, photographed the day we bought it. The back porch had just fallen off.

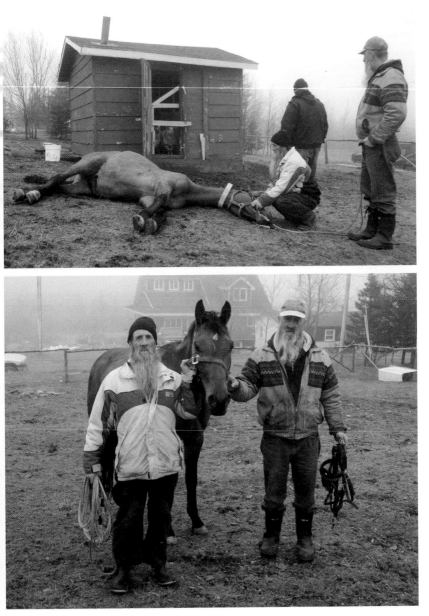

Before and after successful surgery: two clients and their horse (and sheep).

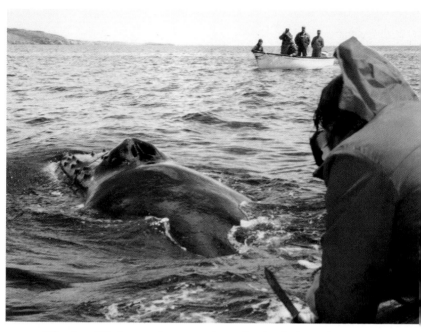

The first EKG ever done on a humpback whale in the ocean.

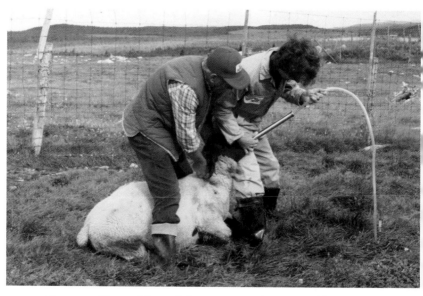

How to relieve a bloated sheep: as gently as possible.

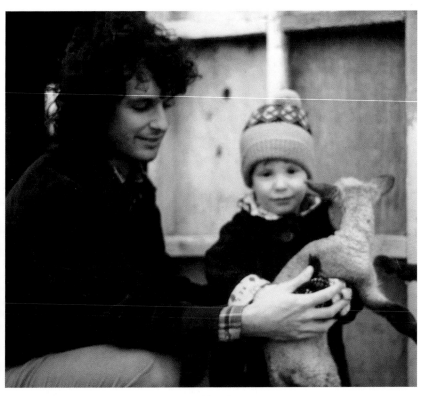

Firstborn: Me and Liam (and lamb).

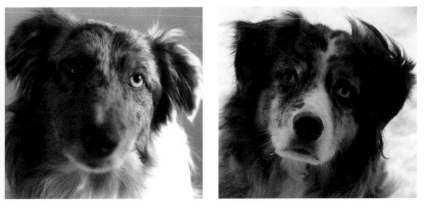

Top dogs: Pogo, cow herder extraordinaire, and Mats, her worthy successor as faithful companion.

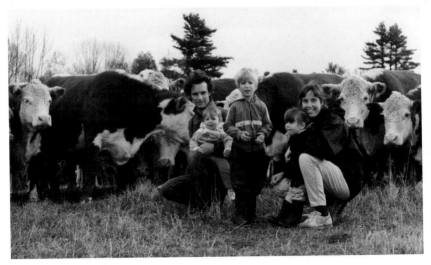

With Astrid, Liam, Adrian and Ingrid and a curious group
of patients.

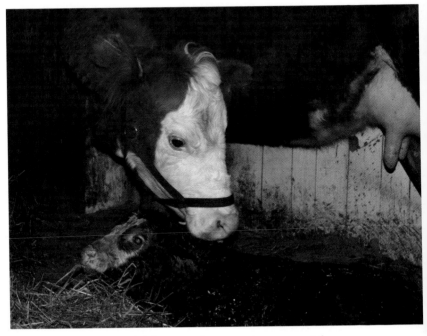

Another special delivery. They are always special.

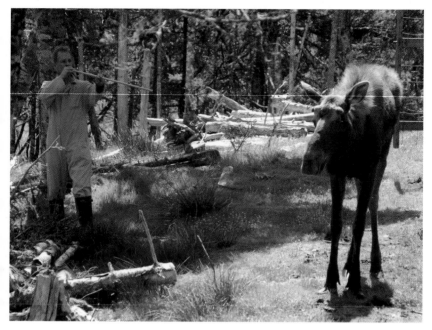

How to trim a moose's hooves: first, place tranquilizing dart in pipe and blow.

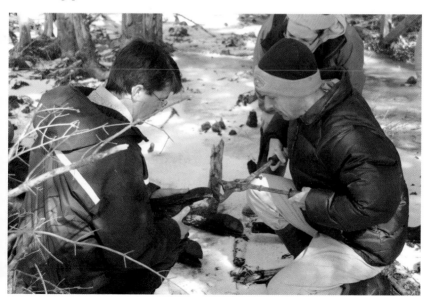

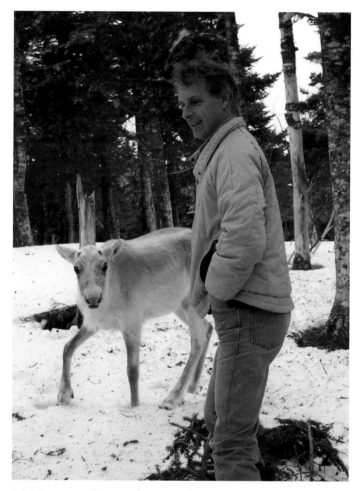
Visiting a resident caribou at Salmonier Nature Park.

20. The Slide

BY THE TIME LIAM WAS SEVEN, his two sisters, Adrian and Astrid, were five and three. Like most mornings, Liam was up before everyone else to draw and had to be pulled away from his latest creation to come to the breakfast table. Adrian stopped running through the house with Mats just long enough to devour a bowl of Corn Flakes. Astrid sat smiling as she placidly watched the excitement of the morning. Once the family was fed, we had to get Liam and Adrian ready for school. Ingrid put together lunches while I searched the house for the crucial page of homework Liam couldn't find.

Outside, freezing rain pelted out of the grey sky and there was a slippery skim on the pavement, so I walked Liam and Adrian to the bus stop. All three of us managed to stay on our feet for the full expedition.

Astrid's babysitter arrived, and after hugs all around, Ingrid, Mats and I left for work.

I spent the first hour answering phone calls in the office and then took a quick trip to a local chicken farm. Even though it was freezing outside, the birds were suffering from overheating. A simple change to the ventilation of the barn brought the temperature down to a healthier level.

When I got back to the office, Sharon handed me a note to call Louise McGurk out near Holyrood.

Mrs. McGurk was worried her cow was dying. "My man's in Alberta and I don't know what to do."

"Can you tell me a little more?"

"She just calved last night, everything looked great, she had a beautiful little calf, but when I came out this morning she was out flat and barely moving. Can you come and see her?"

"What kind of a cow is she, Mrs. McGurk?"

"She's a Jersey, a real darlin', and her calf is beautiful."

"I'll be right out to have a look."

It was a good bet that this was a case of milk fever. The physiological stress of producing milk in unnaturally large quantities is worse in small breeds like Jerseys. These diminutive cows are pushed to make so much milk relative to their body size that they can lose a lot of the calcium they need to keep their bodies healthy and to maintain normal brain activity. Without enough calcium, cattle can get very sick and even die.

Mrs. McGurk's cow needed help fast, and it was normally about an hour's drive from my office to her home in Holyrood. Today, though, I had to balance the urgency of the call with the terrible icy driving conditions. It took me a little over an hour to get to the barn, but I stayed on the road for the full trip.

The McGurk barn was small and neat. Tucked in behind their modern bungalow, it wasn't visible from the road. I gathered up my drug case and carefully picked my way to the barn.

Mrs. McGurk met me at the door. She was a small woman with bright red hair. Her fashionable clothes suggested that she didn't spend much time in the barn. They also didn't hide the fact that she was very pregnant.

"Oh, Doctor, you're here. I'm afraid it may be too late."

The frail Jersey was laid out on her side on the wooden slatted floor. It certainly looked as though she was already dead. But I watched her carefully and could just discern the slow, shallow rise and fall of her ribs. I stepped around to the front of the cow and could see her unseeing and unblinking eyes bulging out of her head.

"It looks like milk fever, Mrs. McGurk. We just might be able to do something for her."

I pulled a bottle of calcium, a length of intravenous tubing and an 18-gauge needle from my case. With such an immobile patient, it was easy to slip the needle into her jugular vein. Once the blood spurted out of the needle, I attached the tubing and the bottle of calcium. I lifted the bottle to the level of my head, and the calcium began flowing down the tube and into the cow's vein.

The calcium worked and it worked fast. After only a few seconds, the Jersey started to blink. Within minutes she lifted her head and looked around. By the time the full bottle had been administered, she was sitting up on her chest.

I pulled the needle from her vein and delivered a second bottle under her skin. The pressure from this injection was obviously uncomfortable, and the cow rose to her feet. She looked around at the needle piercing her side, let out a soft moo and turned to eat her hay.

Mrs. McGurk rubbed her hands over her swollen abdomen. "When this baby comes, I know who I'm callin'. That was a miracle."

There was no argument from me. The treatment of milk fever is truly amazing. It is about as close to magic as we get in vet medicine. It was always a delight to see an animal so sick restored to complete health before your eyes.

The freezing rain had stopped when I went back out to the truck, but the roads were still slick. I took my time driving and arrived home just around suppertime. It felt good to be back, and I looked forward to seeing Ingrid and the kids.

The house was unusually quiet when I stepped inside. I called out, but there was no reply. I found a note on the kitchen counter: "Gone to the hospital, everything's OK."

It was the "everything's OK" part that really worried me. It was unusual for Ingrid to be called out to the hospital, and I wasn't sure why she would have written in those last two words.

Everyone returned home about an hour later, and I heard the story. Ingrid had finished work early and taken the three kids to the grocery store to do some shopping. When they arrived home, Adrian hopped out of the car first and ran to the side of the house. Ingrid saw her slip and fall and then disappear behind the building. When she followed to see where Adrian was, there was no sign of her in the back yard.

Ingrid quickly told Liam to take his youngest sister into the house and then set off to find our missing daughter. The snow in the yard was coated with ice, and even the weight of an adult didn't break through the crust. Ingrid had to pound her feet down with each step in order to stay upright.

Our back yard sits directly on the ocean, and when the kids were small, we had built a picket fence along the edge of the cliff. The previous week, one small section of the fence had blown over in the wind—and Adrian had slipped through that one space. After she had fallen, she slid the full length of the back yard on her stomach like a penguin, through the gap in the fence and out over the edge of the cliff.

Ingrid was horrified to see our daughter lying on the shore nearly thirty feet below. She scrambled down the steep slope and found Adrian lying face down in the one small patch of snow on the rocky shore. Her face was cut, but there didn't seem to be any major damage.

After carrying her back up the hill, Ingrid packed all the kids into the car and drove off to the hospital to make sure there were no broken bones or internal injuries. Thankfully Adrian was fine, and they all had french fries at the hospital cafeteria before returning home.

Two miracles in one day was all that anyone could ask for.

21. Pursuing a Bear

A TWENTY-FOOT BREAKER smashed the bear against the jagged edge of the cliff. He reached out in an attempt to find a foothold as the wave collapsed and carried him back out into the ocean. This was the fourth time he had hit the rock wall and been washed out into the frigid sea.

For twenty-seven days the huge white male had travelled south from Labrador on an ice floe. His temporary refuge had started in the Far North as a flat berg the size of a large church. By the time the currents had taken him to the south end of Newfoundland, the ice was no bigger than a transport truck. When he saw land two miles off his dissolving island, he decided it was time to swim.

Two miles of open ocean was no great test for a skilled swimmer like an adult polar bear, but getting onto the land was proving a definite challenge.

The fifth time the bear was carried to the edge of dry land, he kicked hard with his powerful hind legs just as the water crested at the cliff. With a dull thud he hit the rocks just above the water and drove his nails into cracks in the granite. This time the water washed away without the bear. Once he was free from the grip of the sea, he started climbing.

He made steady progress twenty feet up from his hard

landing to the top of the cliff, looked down at the water, shook himself once and started to run inland.

The bear was first sighted by a young couple walking a section of the East Coast Trail. They watched in amazement as the immense animal was smashed against the rocks over and over. Just when it seemed he would drown from the battering and exhaustion, they saw him climb up toward the trail. Like the bear, they ran. Fortunately, they picked a different direction.

There are two animals in nature that will preferentially hunt humans: the Bengal tiger and the polar bear. I only had the opportunity of looking after one Bengal tiger during my practice. The unauthorized animal was seized from a private zoo and housed at Salmonier Nature Park until a more appropriate permanent residence was found. Polar bears were by comparison common visitors to my part of North America.

The couple on the trail made it quickly back to their car and soon phoned the Wildlife Department with the news that they had seen a yellow polar bear. Wildlife workers tend to be wary of calls from the public, who can be unreliable witnesses where unusual creatures are concerned. But apparently the tipoff that a polar bear sighting is legitimate is the use of the word *yellow*. If a bear is described as white and as big as a van, it's likely a dog.

The southern shore in Newfoundland is not densely populated, but a bear running through the country will likely eventually end up seeing someone. This bear saw his first Newfoundlanders in a bingo hall in Trepassy.

Because the bingo players were facing away from the front door, the man calling numbers was the first to spot the yellow visitor. He had reached into the plastic ball for a number and was straightening up with the microphone in his hand.

"And this time it's under the B— WHOA, there's a friggin' bear in here!"

The patrons turned and screamed in perfect unison. The din from the collective shriek and banging of overturning chairs and tables startled the bear. He fled into the darkness.

Looking for some peace, the bear hurled himself through the picture window of a nearby house. Inside the living room he sat and shook the shards of glass from his body. Thinking he had found a quiet and safe refuge from the madness he had encountered, he rested.

Meanwhile in the basement, the man of the house had turned his attention from watching the Maple Leafs being trounced again to the problem of where that sound of shattering glass had come from. He grabbed his shotgun from the cabinet next to the television and jammed a shell into the breech. It took him four steps to clear the stairs. As he opened the door from the basement, he saw the bear sitting in the living room.

Just as he raised the gun to his shoulder, his wife appeared at the kitchen door at the opposite end of the living room. Seeing the demolished window, the huge bear and her husband pointing his rifle directly at her, she screamed.

The bear, growing tired of all this noise everywhere, left the house the same way he had entered.

When the first call had come in, the local Wildlife dispatcher had called the duty conservation officer. Polar bear sightings were never taken lightly, so the officer was already in his truck when more calls came in about the bingo hall incident. By the time the bear had visited the neighbours' house, the officer was almost in the village.

At the bingo hall the officer was surprised to see that play was in full swing. A couple of patrons with nearly full cards had insisted that the game resume once the chairs and tables were put back in place. Now the officer was politely asked to wait for the current game to finish before he asked any questions. Meanwhile, the presence of the Wildlife truck brought out the man and woman from next door with their breathless explanation of the bear's adventure in their house.

Realizing that the bear was close at hand and a confrontation was likely, the officer phoned for assistance and settled in for a cup of coffee while he watched a few bingo games. When the help arrived, the two men set off in their truck.

It took them two hours to find the bear, sitting quietly at the edge of a copse of alder about thirty yards off a quiet road five miles outside the village.

The men left the truck running in case a quick retreat was called for. The first out of the truck carried a tranquilizer gun and his partner a twelve-gauge semi-automatic shotgun, in case of an emergency. The officers slowly approached to within thirty yards of the bear. The one with the tranquilizer gun knelt and fired a dart loaded with a fast-acting anaesthetic directly into the large muscles of the bear's hind leg.

The startled bear rose on his hind legs, looked directly at the men, dropped to all fours and shuffled away. Within five minutes he was stumbling, and shortly after he was down. The officers recognized the licking motions he was making as usual for this drug and carefully approached the bear.

The officers' truck was towing a culvert trap, a fifteen-foot-long section of steel culvert on wheels with one end solidly barred and the other closed by a triggered wire-mesh door. When they were satisfied the polar bear was safely anaesthetized, they loaded the animal into the trap.

My call came early the next morning. Wildlife told me they had a polar bear in a culvert trap at the park and they wondered if I would be interested in having a look before it was moved. Opportunities to work with these wonderful animals are not common, and in no time I was in my truck and on my way.

A fine crowd of people had gathered at the park by the time I arrived. The two conservation officers were sitting in the parking lot with warm cups of coffee, four staff from the park had come in, and a bear biologist from Labrador who happened to be in the area had dropped by. The bear was standing up in the back of the culvert trap still hitched to the truck.

Polar bears are unimaginably strong. I have seen a bear take a swat at the piece of solid rebar that serves as a trigger for the trap and fold it against the edge of the trap as if it were a paper clip. I could never understand why the bears never ripped their way through the traps when they are clearly more than capable.

The biologist wanted measurements and samples from the bear, and I felt it would be helpful to have a good look at the animal before he was released, so we decided to tranquilize the bear one more time. This time we used a less traumatic method than the explosive dart used by the officers in the field. I loaded a regular syringe with the same tranquilizer and, reaching in through a port in the side of the cage, injected the bear by hand.

Once the bear was down, I quickly went over him to check his condition. He was in marvellous shape and had suffered no apparent external injuries from his long trip south. However, when I looked in his mouth, I found both of his large canine teeth were ground down to the level of the teeth around them, exposing the inner dental pulp and sensitive nerves.

Bears' teeth are critical to their survival. They need them for killing and eating their prey. I was worried that this damage to the animal's teeth could end up causing him serious problems after he was released.

I called my local dentist's house to see if he would be interested in an unusual job. One of his children answered that he was out of the province and would not be home for a few days. I started calling dentists in St. John's. I could offer no compensation, but I thought someone would jump at the opportunity to have a wonderful story to tell their grandchildren. After speaking with five busy or uninterested dentists, I gave up.

The bear had his physical and he'd been measured and sampled. He was ready for a trip back to the Far North. The two conservation officers who had first darted him were to drive the trap to the far north end of the province. We spoke to representatives from the coast guard, and it was soon arranged that a helicopter doing a routine patrol would ferry the bear out to the ice.

Just before the truck left, a phone call came in from a woman on a reserve in central Newfoundland. She claimed to be able to talk to bears and asked if she could see the bear and tell it not to come back south. We all agreed that this either was a good idea or at least would do no harm. The truck left without further delay.

My dentist returned my call that night and told me that a colleague of his in the far north of the province was interested in seeing the bear. This second dentist had a friend who had seen a similar case in a polar bear in Manitoba. He consulted with his friend and was ready for the bear when it arrived.

The bear was put to sleep one more time for the dentist to work on his teeth. The dentist had expected to do a root canal, but after assessing the teeth, he decided to put in deep fillings.

After the bear, his teeth now nearly as good as new, was safely helicoptered out to the ice off Labrador, I reflected on what a successful example of co-operation this whole affair had been. I didn't claim any overtime for seeing the bear; it had been an absolute privilege to be involved. The dentist had not even charged for the materials he'd used, and the coast guard had taken the bear out to the ice on a flight they would have made anyway, bear or no bear.

Our efforts were not universally appreciated, however. A local radio station received a number of calls complaining that the government was now paying for dentistry on bears when many citizens of the province couldn't afford to have their own teeth looked at properly.

Soon after this I heard complaints that the dentist who had done the procedure was practising veterinary medicine without a licence. All I could do was explain that the man was assisting me and working under my licence and remote supervision.

Oblivious to all this fuss, a polar bear hauled himself out of the water and onto a floe of ice off the coast of Labrador, safely home and with reconditioned teeth.

22. A Puck to the Foot

ONCE A WEEK, I had the chance to go down to the local arena and spend an hour playing hockey. For the first ten years, I played in the Carbonear rec league. "Rec" is short for recreation, but it could just as accurately have been spelled "wreck." The league had four teams, referees and a schedule. The idea was to have fun. Some players were skilled; others did not hesitate to use the boards to help them stay upright. The fitness level ranged from a few who could skate all night, to one who carried a pack of cigarettes in his hockey pants so he could have energy-renewing puffs between shifts. There were no slapshots and no bodychecking.

In the beginning, the games were friendly and fun. But it only takes one or two characters who think they are still in the running to be picked for professional glory to change things around. Our league did attract a few of these sorts, and their influence soon led to rough play, hard feelings and eventually a couple of on-ice fights. This new spin on the game had no appeal for me, and I decided my hockey career was through.

The next winter, I was invited to join a bunch that got together once a week for a more friendly game, and I ended up playing some of the most enjoyable sports I'd ever been involved with. Every Tuesday night we would all drive up to the arena in Harbour Grace. Snowstorms that closed the schools all day couldn't keep us away from the rink. We usually had about enough for two teams, and teams were chosen by everyone picking a blue or a white poker chip out of an old velveteen bag that had once contained a bottle of whisky.

Hockey's a fairly safe sport when it's played the way we played it, but there is always the possibility of injury. One night my skates weren't as sharp as they should have been and I ended up falling back on my head after a near collision with one of my opponents. When I first got to my feet, my legs buckled and my vision wasn't as sharp as it had been minutes before. The fact that I couldn't really remember how or why I had fallen, and my teammates' remarking on how far my head had bounced, should have tipped me off that I had a minor concussion. The night's lesson was to never trust someone with a head injury to let you know how badly they have been hurt. Without much sense, I decided that the blurred vision and ringing in my ears were mere trifles and played the rest of the night. Luckily I had no long-term effects from the fall, but it could have easily been more serious.

The only other injury I suffered was the night Clarence hit me in the foot with a shot. Clarence was a retired police officer who faithfully turned up for games. As a player, he did his best work on banjo and mandolin at our Christmas parties.

In hockey, standing in front of the net can be a dangerous pastime. In higher levels of the game, players can fire that hard bit of rubber toward you at around a hundred miles an hour. I had no worry about those speeds with our group.

The night of the injury, I was trying to keep players on the other team away from the front of our goal when the puck came back to Clarence on the blue line. He raised his stick and shot at the net. The puck didn't move much faster than a quick skater could.

I stopped the puck. Unfortunately, I stopped it using that small section on the inside of a skate where there's a thin fabric gap in the armour. I felt a sharp pain and was immediately unable to put my foot to the ice without great agony.

There are few as foolish as middle-aged hockey players. We don't have the sense to pace ourselves during games and we never seem to know when we should quit. Despite all the pain and not being much help to the team, I played out the game. Driving home was torture, and I limped into the house and directly to bed.

By chance Ingrid wasn't working the next morning, and she drove me to the hospital for an X-ray. There were no fractures.

Back home, my foot wasn't feeling any better. I still couldn't bear to put it to the ground. It was going to be impossible to do any vet work if I couldn't walk or drive, so at least I could look forward to a couple of days off work.

But first I checked my answering machine. There was one call. Norm Molly, from Molly's Road just down from the hospital, had a goat kidding. I called Norm up and his wife answered.

"Norm's in the barn, he's got one kid out and the next one must be stuck."

"I'll be there right away." Click.

What did I just say? My foot was killing me and I could hardly stand.

Next I heard from Ingrid. "What did you just say?"

"Well, Norm's goat is having trouble getting a kid out, and he's a good guy, and if he has to wait for the vet from St. John's to come out he'll lose the kid . . . and my foot's not that bad."

"So you think you can drive the truck and get to the barn and deliver a kid?"

"Well, actually I was thinking that since you were off today, you might like to see some animals, a good chance to see some cute newborn kids . . . Maybe you could come along and give me a hand."

Ingrid gave me a variety of incredulous looks, but soon I was in the passenger seat of the truck and we were on our way to Norm's. It was a short drive, and before long we were stopped at the end of a narrow lane off a back road. The only clue that there was any kind of farming in the area was the small red barn out behind Norm's house.

The wind howled and the sky was a uniform grey as I cautiously stepped down from the cab. I hobbled along the side of truck, opened the side door and hauled out my obstetrical case. Ingrid hurried to my side and mercifully offered to carry the case for me.

Now I had time to notice that the area between the truck and Norm's barn was a solid sheet of ice. The night before it had rained and then frozen. Anywhere that the rainwater had collected was now like glass. It would be a challenge even with a good set of legs to get to the barn without ending up with a tumble or two, but with an aching foot, this was going to be interesting.

Norm came sliding across the space between his house and the truck. He was dressed in a snowmobile suit that had seen better days and a threadbare Montreal Canadiens cap. His perpetual smile left him with creases from the corners of his eyes and prominent red cheeks.

"Morning, Norm," I said. "Would you mind carrying this case to the barn for me, please?" And then in a quieter voice, "Ingrid, can you help me across this ice?"

Norm grabbed the case and made his way quickly toward the barn. He slipped violently a couple of times but managed to bring his feet under himself quickly enough to stay upright. Obviously this wasn't his first time across this treacherous path.

I took Ingrid's arm for support and the two of us carefully tottered across the yard. It wasn't pretty; we looked like an old couple who really shouldn't be allowed out alone for this kamikaze constitutional. But we eventually made it.

Norm's barn looked more like a shed with a smaller shed stuck on the side. But it was red like a barn and it had been painted quite recently. The entrance was made up of two doors; the outer one was heavy and well fastened. Even the winds of Newfoundland weren't going to disturb the inhabitants. Inside, a number of bare lights hung from the ceiling and somehow there was no dust on the bulbs. It was bright and cheery.

Along one side was an aisle with pens and goats in every one. Goats are eternally curious, and our entrance brought everyone up on their back legs. Well, almost everyone. From a pen near the middle of the barn came a pathetic bleating.

Norm opened the small door to the pen and dragged out a desperate-looking nanny goat. Her eyes were listless, and she panted between her pitiable groans. Beside her, a newborn kid stumbled around trying out his new legs. He shook his head, flopping his ears from side to side as he tried to understand why his mother wouldn't co-operate with his efforts to get his first drink.

"Norm, I'll need some soap and warm water for this, if you don't mind, and it would be great if you had something for me to sit on while I work. My foot isn't the best."

"We're all ready for you, Doc." Norm went just down the aisle to the abandoned freezer where he stored his feed and came back with a pink section of towel neatly ripped into a square and folded around a bar of soap still inside its wrapper. "And here's your water." He hauled over a white plastic bucket and lifted its red lid to reveal warm clean water.

"That's real service, Norm. I don't often get things as nice as this."

"How would this do for a seat?" Norm upended another large plastic pail with a clean bottom.

"Perfect! Let's get to work."

I sat on the improvised stool and leaned in to take a look at my patient. She was tired but still able to stand, and was making weak and ineffective pushes. Most likely she had another kid stuck inside and was worn out from trying to move it.

The water and soap were put to good use as I carefully washed my hands and arms. Even in a tidy barn it's important to stay as clean as possible during deliveries. I pressed my fingers together to form a cone shape and slowly pushed my hand into the birth passage. Once my hand was inside a little past the wrist, I felt a hoof and a leg, then another, and then another. Three feet coming. Either this was a contortionist on its way out or we had another two kids. I took one of the legs between my thumb and index finger and slowly followed it along until I came to a chest. From there I moved across to the other leg attached to this body and felt my way back to the foot. Now I knew which two legs belonged to the same kid.

I took the remaining leg in my fingers and again felt along it until I came to another chest. This time I put my fingers together and pushed the chest of the second kid farther back into the birth canal. Once the kid was over the brim of the mother's pelvic bones, I could feel him or her slip back down into the uterus.

From this point the delivery was more straightforward. After a light tug on the remaining two legs, I pushed in farther with my hand, gently cupped it around the unborn kid's head and was able to pull the kid forward to the point where the birth canal narrowed into the cervix. The kid's head and my hand wouldn't both fit through this space, though. My options were to pull on the legs and see whether the head would come the right way or to put a snare around the kid's head to guide it in the right direction.

My approach to treating animals, especially when assisting deliveries, was generally to try the simplest, least invasive technique first. A snare for delivering kids or lambs is a clever and helpful tool. It is simply a small loop of plastic-coated wire threaded through a plastic guide tube. The idea is to put the snare around the kid's head and push the plastic guide up under the animal's chin. You then tighten the snare to the point where it won't squeeze on the neck or slip over the head. When the snare is in place, a tug on the apparatus pulls on the kid's head by putting pressure on the back of the neck. This simple device has saved many lives.

This time I decided to first try pulling without the snare. As I firmly pulled on the legs, the kid moved forward. Soon its nose was visible, and with a final tug, his head popped out into the world. More gentle pressure brought the rest of the body out.

The kid shook his head and let out his first bawl. Normally the mother would respond immediately to this call and begin cleaning off her newborn, but this poor goat didn't care much about the kid. She was tired and she no doubt sensed that her work wasn't over.

I took a bottle of iodine from my case and spilled a little over the broken end of the umbilical cord. Norm lifted the kid to the front of the mother ("Congratulations, ma'am, you're the mother of a bouncing baby buck") to see if she would start to clean him off. She still didn't show any interest, so Norm set to work with a towel.

It was back to work for me. I washed up again and pushed my arm inside for another feel around. This time the usual two front feet and a head were coming in the right direction. This kid was a little smaller, and this size difference, combined with the fact that the nanny's insides had just been stretched, allowed me to pull it out with my hand cupped over his head. Despite his size, this fellow was even louder than his brother. The mother goat, seeming to sense her ordeal was over, turned her head and answered.

We moved the last kid up in front of her and she started sniffing him all over. She let out a couple more contented-sounding bleats and started cleaning him off. It always amazed me how clean and dry a goat can make a kid just with her tongue.

After drinking a bucket of warm water, the mother regained more of her strength and interest. Although the other two kids were dried off, we moved them up to her face to encourage some bonding of the family. I had Norm fetch a little goat feed from his freezer and sprinkle it on the two kids to encourage their mother to lick them. Soon we had a close-knit family of four. The future looked fine for this bunch.

I always liked to give new families like this a little time to themselves, so I suggested to Norm that we should all leave.

As Norm turned out the lights, Ingrid took my arm, and I left the warmth of the barn for one more limping crossing of the ice to the truck.

23. Impaled

MY JOB WAS ALWAYS a great source of entertainment for visitors. My father particularly enjoyed accompanying me on calls when he came to visit, and I found him an ideal travelling companion. He had started his career as a high school principal, but retired early to farm the family homestead. He was an experienced and intelligent workmate.

My parents often visited in the middle of the summer, a time when most animals were on pasture and at their healthiest, so it was a slower time of year for my work.

A call from Albert saying that one of his sheep was having trouble lambing coincided with one summer visit from my mother and father. Albert was a retired scientist who had taken up sheep farming. Farming with Albert was a scientific affair: every problem could be studied up and reasoned out. His farm featured many interesting and unusual innovations, complex ideas that at times seemed to ignore farming tradition and involved a certain amount of wheel re-inventing.

Dad and I left for Albert's place near Placentia early in the morning. It was a beautiful warm day, and I was confident that we would deliver the lamb and have a leisurely visit with plenty of time for farming theories and discussion of politics.

As we parked the truck outside Albert's barn, I saw him coming out the side door drying his arms with a towel. He was a tall man, and with his neat clothes and impeccable posture he cut an impressive figure.

"It seems we've run into a little dystocia here," he informed me. "From what I can ascertain, there are two youngsters attempting to be born at the same time."

"Okay, let's have a look."

The three of us trooped into the barn together, where I found that Albert had assembled all the materials that I would need for the delivery. The ewe having the problems was in a separate pen in a room with a smooth concrete floor. Just outside the pen, a bucket of sudsy water and a neat pile of towels were ready.

A pair of legs were protruding from the sheep's back end, and her grunts and straining made it clear she wasn't happy.

"How long has this been going on, Albert?"

"As I usually do, I had a quick look at all the animals before breakfast. At that time, I didn't notice any of the flock in any particular distress. However, after breakfast I found this little lady straining over in the corner by herself. I did a vaginal exam, and when it seemed that her problems were a little beyond my abilities, I gave you a call."

After washing and lubricating my arm, I reached up inside my patient to see what the problem was. With a careful feel around the inside of the mother's uterus, I determined that two lambs were competing for the status of first-born.

Deliveries of lambs are quite different from those of calves. With calves, the newborn often weighs a hundred pounds or more, and the hulking mother is capable of bruising the arms of anyone trying to come between the two of them. Calf deliveries require skill and finesse, but often a certain amount of brute force too. Sheep are more delicate creatures; a lamb delivery requires a subtle touch. Too much force can damage both the mother and the lambs.

Sheep often have twins or even triplets, and normally, one lamb is delivered first while its sibling waits patiently farther back in the uterus. Occasionally, though, the lambs will line up inside in such a way that all their legs start moving to the outside together. Of course there isn't enough room for two lambs to pass together through the bony opening formed by the pelvis, and trouble results.

After I determined that the legs we were seeing in this case belonged to two different lambs, my first step was to move everyone back inside. The sheep always feels that this move is counterproductive and of course resists the backwards movement of the lambs.

With my hand still inside the mother's uterus, I carefully ran my fingers along the legs until I determined which belonged to each lamb. Next, I chose the lamb that was farthest forward to be delivered first. The legs of the other I gently pushed to the back of the uterus and out of the way. Now I placed the first lamb into a normal lambing position, with the front legs stretched out and the head up. Once the front legs were outside, I pulled on them gently with my other hand. Simultaneously, with the hand inside I made sure the head stayed in a position that wouldn't catch on the rim of the pelvis.

In short order the first lamb was out, but right away we realized it wasn't breathing. Disappointments and heartbreak are common in farming, and this was just one more instance.

Deep inside, every vet knows that calls like this are not the complete disasters that they appear to be on the surface. Even the delivery of dead lambs can be a partial success if the mother survives. Without help, a sheep unable to deliver will most certainly die.

I had no time for these thoughts as I gave all my attention to the lamb still inside. We all held our breaths as the legs and head of the second lamb emerged with a gentle push from its mother. After a few agonizing seconds, the newborn shook its head, blinked its eyes and snorted. The atmosphere in the barn lightened rapidly.

We gave the lamb a vigorous rub with some hay, put a little iodine on his navel and moved him to the front of his mother. Immediately she changed from an exhausted, uninterested rag to a bright and proud mother. Mother and child called to each other. The mother stimulated her newborn with a rough full-body grooming, and he unsteadily lifted his head.

Once we had cleaned up, Albert suggested we have a cup of tea down at his house. By the time we were halfway there from the barn, Dad and Albert were deep in conversation. My father asked about the varieties of hay that Albert planted, and Albert started into a long description of the pros and cons of all the types he had considered. Dad was quick to suggest three more that might be appropriate. I anticipated that I would be mostly listening during this tea break.

A cozy fire was burning in the wood stove, and I reflected

on how pleasant this visit was going to be. Before Albert put the kettle on, he looked over at his phone, where the answering machine was blinking. He flipped on the machine, and we all heard my secretary saying that I should phone the office ASAP. I called Sharon back and asked her what the problem was.

"You better get over to Mike Turner's right away. He's got a horse with a real bad wound. He said something about a rail driven into its chest."

I asked Sharon to call Mike and tell him I was on my way.

"Sorry, Albert," I said, "but we have to run off on an urgent call. We'll take a rain check on the tea."

"That's unfortunate. I would have liked to explain to your father about the different genotypes of grass and the reasons why the one I'm using is superior."

I quickly wrote up a bill for Albert, and Dad and I scrambled out to the truck.

"It's too bad we didn't have time for tea," my dad said. "I would have liked to explain to that guy about the alternative types of grass available. He was missing some of the better ones."

No doubt it would have been an interesting talk, but for now we had to rush off to see a horse in Shearstown that apparently had something driven into its chest. We drove quickly and arrived at Mike's place in a little over a half-hour. A crowd of his family was milling around.

As we stopped the car I pointed out a large red-faced man in bib overalls waving his arms wildly in the air. "That's Mike," I told my dad.

As soon as we opened the doors we could hear him as well as see him.

"You @#$% moron! Why in the @#$& did you run this #$%!@# horse into that #$@% fence?"

"Mornin', Mike."

"What? Oh, hi, Doc. We've got a @#$% mess this morning. Hey! Get that @#$% 'arse into the #$%!@ barn, ya moron."

"Mike, this is my father. He's visiting from Ontario."

"How are ya, skipper? Will you get that @#$% 'arse into the @#$*% barn, ya blood of a bitch?"

"Bite me, old man!"

This reply came from Mike's son, Mike Junior, who had been the brunt of Mike's verbal barrage to this point. Although slim and attired in ripped jeans and an AC/DC T-shirt, he was in some matters very much like Mike Senior.

"You lazy son of a bitch, get that 'arse in there before I rings yer @#$%* neck. So is this yer first time on the island, skipper?"

I don't think my father was used to this kind of language, but he didn't miss a beat. "No, I've been here quite a few times before."

"I hope you're enjoying your visit. It's been a peach of a summer so far. Will you get off your lazy !@#$% ass and move that !@#$% 'arse!"

"!@#$ off, old man!"

After all of this fuss and profanity being expended to move the horse, it was a little awkward to explain that I really didn't want to examine her in the dark barn.

"Mike, I'd actually prefer to have a look at your horse out here in the sun."

"No trouble, me old cock. Hey! Get that !@#$% 'arse out here for the vet to see."

"You've been runnin' yer yap at me for a half an hour to move the *&%$# thing into the barn!"

"I don't give a #$!@. Get the !@#$% out here."

Finally the horse was brought out to the flat stretch of gravel in front of the barn, and Mike Senior and Junior took a break from their verbal battle.

The horse had indeed been stabbed in the chest. A cylindrical piece of wood nearly a foot long and four inches in diameter protruded from the front of the animal just inside the leg.

I hoped that the stick was only in a short distance. If so, this shouldn't be too serious.

"Mike, could you hold the horse while I see if I can pull that out?"

Mike pulled his thumbs out of the straps of his overalls and spat a wad of chewing tobacco on the ground. He waddled over and took a firm grip on the animal's halter. Once I saw that he had a solid grip, I took hold of the end of the stick and gave a short tug.

It didn't move. At least it didn't move relative to the horse. The pressure I had put on the stick obviously caused a jolt of pain, and the horse reared up and lashed out with her front legs. I was positioned directly in the middle of the horse's chest, and the legs sailed past my head on both sides, missing me by inches. The left leg didn't continue forward—it found resistance when it smacked up against Mike's shoulder. The force of the blow spun Mike around and rolled him a short distance across the gravel.

Mike Junior took great delight in this turn of events. "Old man, can't you 'old an 'arse?"

"You !@#$% *&#$@!, I'll hold your !@#$% head in a minute."

"I'd like to see you, old man. You can't do squat."

Although this repartee did have a certain charm, I really wanted to get another chance to remove this stick and see how much damage it had caused. While the Mikes continued sparring, I considered how I should best proceed with my procedure.

The horse was now beyond reasoning with. She was likely panicked from the moment this small log had stabbed into her. The wild atmosphere provided by the owners and our attempt to move the stick had certainly made matters worse. My choices were to wrench the stick out quickly and have things over with, or to load the horse up with painkillers before proceeding.

The painkillers would take some of the edge off the horse's demeanour, but I could see that administering an intravenous drug was going to be nearly as stressful to her as pulling out the stick. I decided to make one last attempt.

The Mikes had momentarily forgotten about the horse and were over by the barn door insulting each other in increasingly loud voices.

"Hey, guys, come over here!" I called.

Both stopped in mid-sentence.

"Look, this horse is really spooked and I'm going to need both of you to hold on to her while I pull out the stick. Do you think the two of you can hold her down?"

"My son there isn't a !@#$% horse born that the two of us couldn't— . . ."

"That's great. Now you just stay here while I get the grin."

I ran back to the truck to fetch the grin, or twitch. This short loop of chain on the end of a three-foot stick is used to twist a horse's nose. Surprisingly, the result of this manoeuvre is not pain but rather relaxation. Some suggest that the twisting of the horse's nose results in a release of pain-reducing endorphins.

Mike and Mike held tightly to the halter as I placed the chain loop around the horse's nose and tightened it. Once the grin was firmly in place, I handed the base of the instrument to the senior Mike and asked him to hold it tightly against the side of the horse's head.

The horse relaxed noticeably, and I was able to get a good look at the stick. From the way it moved when the horse shifted her weight from leg to leg, I could tell that it was deeply imbedded.

"Okay, guys, hang on tight—I'm going to give this a yank."

"Giv'er, Doc."

I pulled much harder than the first time, but still the stick didn't budge. The grin, however, was doing its job. The horse hardly moved this time.

I asked the Mikes to keep holding while I went to the truck for more equipment and ideas. As I rummaged around inside, my father asked if I thought maybe something might be sticking out the side of the stick, holding it in place. This hadn't occurred to me but it made perfect sense. I grabbed a long set of forceps and returned to the horse.

"How ya doin', guys?"

"Perfect," they replied in unison.

I asked Mike Senior to apply a little more pressure to the grin, and then I slid the forceps in alongside the stick and then around its circumference. In about six inches, I felt a metallic resistance. I pushed the flesh away, and now I could see what was keeping the stick in place. A nail protruded from the stick, its pointed end angled toward me. Each time I had pulled, I was raking this nail through tissue.

I carefully placed the forceps over the back of the nail and pushed the stick in slightly as I closed the forceps, pushing down on the nail and pressing it close against the stick. By slightly prying out the tissue in front of the nail, I was then able to gently slide the stick out. It was over two feet long.

It astonished me that a stake this size hadn't proved fatal. It had somehow missed the heart and the many large and important blood vessels coursing through the impaled part of the body.

Mike Senior nodded to his son as we examined the stick. "Nice work, my son."

"We held her on, old man."

We kept the grin in place as I cleaned the wound as best I could and stuffed the hole with iodine-soaked gauze. Once the grin was removed, the horse moved off to a section of grass against the barn and started to eat. It looked likely she would suffer no serious after-effects.

In short order, I injected her with a dose of penicillin and tetanus toxoid, wrote up the bill and left instructions for further treatment of the patient.

With the work all done, I was still curious to know how this long stick with a nail in it had managed to be driven that far into the horse.

"So how did this happen, Mike?"

"Me and the young fella were bringin' the cattle in from the pasture and one of them gave him a jaysus of a kick. So bright arse here picks up a stick and starts chasin' after the one that booted him. The !@#$% moron runs the cow right up to the horse and the horse rears up and comes down on a piece of the fence."

"I'd like to see what you'd do if that cow kicked *you*, old man."

"You're a !@#$% idiot."

I had really had enough of this for one day. "Gotta go, guys. Give me a call if you have any trouble with the horse."

Safely back in the truck, I asked my dad what he had thought of the Mikes.

"Oh they're all right. But I'd really like to straighten out that Albert guy about his choice of grass."

24. The Child's Decision

FRIDAY NIGHTS I SET ASIDE for dogs and cats. There was enough work with cows and horses during the day, and time with the family was an important priority, so I never attended to more than a handful of pets in an evening.

Generally, I saw dogs and cats for routine health checks, vaccinations and dewormings. If animals had medical problems, I would do what I could with my simple facilities in the small clinic I built across the road from our house and refer complicated cases to small-animal practices in St. John's. Working alone, I was limited in my surgeries to castrations, spays and straightforward trauma cases.

One Friday evening, I had seen a puppy with mild diarrhea and vaccinated two cats and three dogs. I was ready to close up the clinic when an expensive-looking car sped into the drive. I watched as a young couple and a small boy jumped from the car and ran toward the clinic. The man cradled a blood-soaked bundle of sheets in his arms.

I put down the bottle of disinfectant I was using to clean the exam table and opened the door to the waiting room to meet the new arrivals. The man and woman looked to be in their early thirties. The clothes they wore marked them as well off. The woman had tears in her eyes and began speaking as soon as she stepped inside.

"We only opened the door for a second and she got out. She went straight for the road and the first car went right over her." She shuddered heavily and wiped her reddened eyes with the sleeve of her coat.

"Come on in and we'll see what we can do."

The mother turned to her son and placed both hands on his shoulders. "Can you wait out here, Nick, while Dad and I go in and get Susie fixed up?"

"Sure, Mom, I'm okay."

I ushered the parents into the examining room with their burden of injured cat. "Let's just have a look at Susie and see what's going on." I took the wrapped cat from the man's arms and placed it on the examining table. I heard a weak and piteous meow as I folded back the sheets. It didn't take me long to assess the seriousness of the situation.

The car had driven directly over the cat's back end, and the abdominal wall was burst open. The back was crushed so badly that it felt like rough sand in a bag, and when I touched her there, there was no pain response. Both back legs were broken into dozens of shards and dangled at unnatural angles. The cat was in shock but not showing signs of great pain or panic.

I stepped back and paused. It was never easy to tell owners when an animal was irreparably injured.

"I'm afraid," I told them, "that Susie is hurt pretty bad."

The woman turned her back and sobbed. The man put his arms around her for a moment and then came back to the edge of the table.

"What can you do for her, Doctor?"

"I'm sorry, but there really isn't anything we can do for an injury this bad. Susie is suffering, and the only humane thing we can do is to put her to sleep."

The woman's sobbing moved up to hysterical weeping. Between her tears she snuffled and managed to say, "I never should have opened that door."

The man put both hands on the table and leaned toward me. "Isn't there *anything* you can do?"

I had seen this kind of sorrow and guilt in owners many times before. It was going to take some time and compassion before this could be helped in the only way possible.

I spent a long time with the man delicately going over the extent of the poor animal's injuries. With the description of each part of the damage, he continued to insist that there had to be some way to deal with that particular problem. My relentless account of the severity of the mutilation and the hopelessness of the situation eventually wore him down.

"Okay, we'll put Susie down." He blurted these words out before turning away and weeping as uncontrollably as his wife. The two of them embraced, and their sobs slowly abated in unison. I felt like an intruder on this private moment of grief, but I knew that as horrific as my suggestion seemed, it was the only way to help poor Susie.

The man let go of his wife and turned back to face me. He wiped the back of his hand across his eyes and briskly rubbed both hands down his thighs. "Okay, okay. Here's what we're going to do," he said. "We'll call Nick in, and you tell him that you're going to see what you can do for Susie. Give us about ten minutes to get home, then give us a call and tell us that she didn't make it."

I had never been given a suggestion quite like this before, and it immediately struck me as a very wrong approach. It was always my feeling that honesty would never get you in trouble if you were sincere in your efforts. Lies and misinformation have a tendency to pile up problems. I did not like the idea of lying to this child.

"I have a suggestion for how to handle this. How about if you two go out into the waiting room and I have a little talk with Nick in here?"

Their heads snapped around to face each other. They hadn't been expecting this.

"But he's only seven," the mother protested.

"Is Susie Nick's cat?" I asked.

"She is. We got her for him two years ago. He feeds her and cleans out her litter box."

"I think if Nick is old enough to have a cat, he's old enough to be responsible when things go wrong. Let me talk to him. Don't you worry, I'll be careful."

Both parents leaned over Susie and rubbed her across the head. Neither could say anything as they left the examining room.

I followed them to the door. "Hey, Nick, can I talk to you for a minute?"

"Yeah, okay." He put down the comic he was reading and came into the examining room.

I closed the door. "Come over here, Nick, and have a look at Susie. She's smashed up pretty bad, isn't she?"

"Yeah. That's gross."

"You know, Nick, her back is broken, her legs are broken, and she really hurt a lot of things inside. The worst part of all this is that I can't fix these things. They're busted up too badly."

Nick looked up over the side of the table and ran his hand over his injured cat.

"Nick, your cat isn't very happy now, and that's too bad, but you and I can't make her happy."

He looked up at me and asked, "What are we gonna do?"

"Sometimes, Nick, when animals are hurt really bad, the only thing we can do is put them to sleep. It's not a nice thing to do, but we do it for the animals. We don't like seeing them unhappy, and if they can't get better, it's the one thing we can do to help out a bit. What do think we should do with Susie?"

Nick heaved a heavy sigh, but there wasn't a tear in his eye. "I guess we better put her to sleep. I don't want her to be unhappy."

This kid impressed me with his selfless compassion for his cat. He seemed to truly understand what was best for his pet.

"Can you tell your mom and dad about this?"

Nick shrugged. "Sure."

I called his parents back into the waiting room. I said, "Nick wants to tell you something."

"Mom, Dad, we have to put Susie to sleep. She's suffering and we can't make her happy again."

Both parents dissolved into tears and turned away from their son. Nick went over to his mother and put his arms around her waist. "It's okay, Mom. Susie will be happier this way."

Nick's reassurance didn't slow his parents' tears. I don't think anyone was sure exactly what they were crying about. There was the pain of losing the family pet and the relief of having the situation explained to their son. Perhaps more than any of this, there was also pride in the way their young boy had handled such a difficult decision.

25. Where the Caribou Don't Yet Roam

HOW DID I EVER get myself into this?

I was freezing cold and it was all I could do to keep myself inside the box of the speeding pickup truck. My legs were spread so that I was jammed tightly between the spare tire and the sides of the truck. My arms were wrapped around a sleeping caribou, keeping her in a position that allowed her to safely breathe. I wished that I hadn't asked the driver to see how fast we could get to the drop-off point.

Working for the government, I had the opportunity to help out with wildlife projects. This one was a caribou relocation. For various reasons, caribou were plentiful in some parts of the province and not present at all in others. Wildlife officials were always on the lookout for places where the environment was suited to caribou but there was no resident population.

Introducing caribou into those areas was a complex business, requiring a great deal of planning. Healthy animals had to be sourced from herds that would not suffer from their removal. There had to be enough food, water and shelter for the newcomers. The level of threat from predators in the area had to be considered. In rural Newfoundland the worst predators tended to be the two-legged variety. The early stages of a relocation are the most critical, and even small amounts of poaching can doom a project.

This particular relocation had the best approach to poaching that I had ever seen. Before the work began, wildlife officials visited all the local schools and asked them to sponsor individual animals. The students raised some money for the project and chose a name for their caribou, and in some cases school representatives were invited to witness the release of the animal. When the caribou were moved, every one "belonged" to some kids in the area. Filling the barrens with game wardens wouldn't have provided the caribou with more protection from poaching. The most hardened poacher wouldn't risk the scorn of every school-age child in the region.

Once the source of caribou and their new home was decided on, a technique for the actual move had to be chosen.

In Newfoundland, a favourite tool for wildlife work is the helicopter. To capture caribou, two wildlife technicians sit in the back of a helicopter armed with a tranquilizer gun. The pilot flies into an area filled with caribou, an individual target is selected, and the helicopter swoops in. The wildlife technicians will do these jobs only with the very best pilots because of the very technical flying that is required. The pilot tries to position the helicopter a few feet above and just to the side of a bolting caribou. He or she must keep one eye on the animals while watching for trees, rocks and power lines that may suddenly appear.

One of the technicians who is harnessed into the helicopter leans out the door with his pistol and tries to deliver a tranquilizer-filled dart into the large muscles of the hind leg of the running caribou. Once the caribou is hit, the pilot rapidly ascends to a few hundred feet to allow the darted animal to relax. It's a wild ride; after my first trip I learned the nauseating perils of sitting in a backwards-facing seat.

In order to get enough drug to knock down an excited caribou into the small volume offered by a dart, you have to use a very strong drug. Carfentanil, one of the drugs we often used, is considered to be up to forty thousand times as potent as morphine.

If the dart ends up in a large muscle and the drug is properly ejected from the dart, the caribou will stop running, stumble and eventually lie down. Once the animal is lying quietly, the helicopter lands a short distance away and the technicians run over to the anaesthetized caribou. They check the animal to be sure that it is well asleep and that no damage has been done by the dart or from falling. Then they securely tie the caribou to a small metal stretcher and load it into the helicopter. In this particular capture, the helicopter then ferried the caribou to a nearby loading area where pickup trucks were waiting.

This was how I found myself in the back of a pickup truck monitoring a caribou for the hour-long drive to the release site near Western Bay.

The last fifteen minutes of each ride involved a trip over a primitive boulder-strewn road out into the barrens. At the release site, I would first crawl out of the truck, stretch and bang my hands together to try to get some blood and warmth back into my limbs. I would then draw the reversal drug up into a syringe and inject it into a vein in the caribou before the drug froze in the syringe. Within thirty seconds, the reversal drug would take effect—the caribou would blink its eyes, perhaps shake its head once, leap to its feet and run off as if nothing had happened.

By the end of the day we had moved a dozen caribou to their new home. The work was fascinating, but it was also exhausting, bone-chilling and, it seemed to me, far too dangerous. At our meeting to assess the day's work, I suggested that both the animals and the vets would be more comfortable and safe in vehicles with an enclosed back, like a van.

The second day of the move, we changed from pickup trucks to vans with hay spread out in the back. This time the moves were completed in relative comfort. Instead of concentrating on staying inside the truck box and surviving hypothermia, we were able to carefully monitor the breathing, temperature and heart rate of the caribou while an assistant helped keep them upright and comfortable.

Landing a dart in a caribou from a helicopter requires great skill and carries heavy responsibility. The drugs are dangerous, and in the mania of a helicopter chase, everyone must remain as calm as possible to avoid the risk of workers being exposed to them. The smallest pinprick from a needle holding enough drug to knock down a running wild caribou could prove fatal to a person. The potency of the drug made losing a dart unacceptable. The shooters rarely miss, but when they do, the project is put on hold until the dart is found. These potent drugs and the explosive delivery system also present some danger to the darted animal. On the second day of the project, one of the shooters hit a caribou in the chest. The dart penetrated between two ribs and released the drug into the chest cavity. The technicians immediately saw that they had a problem; wounds to the chest can damage the lungs and heart or interfere with breathing by allowing air into the thorax. They pulled the caribou into the helicopter and told the pilot to find one of the vets. The pilot radioed out to the transfer site and was told a vet was in transit in the van. The helicopter set off from the capture site trying to find the vehicle.

The van was driving through the centre of the town of Bay Roberts when we heard the helicopter thunder directly over top of us. Our driver understood something was wrong and pulled over.

With the roar of the engines and the blast of prop wash, the helicopter dropped down on a suburban front lawn. The door of the helicopter flew open and two uniformed men rushed across the lawn with a caribou on a stretcher. We pulled the stricken animal inside the van and propped her up on the hay beside the caribou we were moving. The technicians scrambled back to the helicopter and were soon in the air and returning to the caribou herd. As we pulled away, I glanced out the back window and caught sight of two women staring out their living-room window with their mouths agape.

There was no time to waste. I wanted to get to the release area quickly so that we could administer the antidote as quickly as possible. During the ride I closed the wound with a couple of stitches.

The truck pulled off the highway onto the rough gravel road that led to our treeless and boulder-strewn release site.

When we came to a halt, I carefully checked over the animal. Its breathing was normal and there was no evidence of any damage to ribs or of air escaping around the wound site. The technicians and I pulled the caribou out of the van and set her down on a clump of moss. I slipped the needle into the prominent vein on a front leg and pushed in the reversal agent.

The caribou's quick snort put a cloud of steam in the cold, still air and she bolted to her feet. The procedure was repeated for the second caribou with similar success. We all stood back as the caribou ran off to join the province's newest herd.

26. Soaked

THE WIND HOWLED AS Mats and I got out of the truck and opened the door to my office. The day before had been busy, with a bunch of calves suffering from diarrhea and a long drive to a cow whose uterus had prolapsed. By the time I arrived home after putting her back together, it was well past suppertime.

With all my scheduled calls finished up and this unfriendly weather, there was a good chance I would have a slow day. The office was swarming when I got in. As the chill from the cold weather outside faded, I watched my colleagues scurrying about the office with plates and utensils. The place smelled like bacon.

Dexter, the agricultural representative, poked his head out from the coffee room down the hall. "You havin' some breakfast, Doc?"

I put my drug case down and went over to see what he was up to. Two electric frying pans were hard at work.

"We got eggs, bacon and moose sausages this morning."

"Oh man, I just had breakfast."

Fred, the government road inspector, stepped out of his office and grinned. "You gotta be like the hobbits. This is just secondsies."

The smell of bacon and sausages did, I admit, fill me with temptation. I reasoned that I hadn't had that much breakfast after all, and it wouldn't be right to refuse this offer of a chance to spend some time with my friends. "Let me put my coat away."

When I got back to the coffee room, everyone was settled in around the table for breakfast. Somehow it wouldn't surprise me if more than one of us was there for secondsies. The others were already working their way through piles of bacon, sausage and scrambled eggs. A carton of orange juice sat in the middle of the table. Yet there seemed to be something missing from our normal breakfast get-togethers.

"Where's the bread, guys?" I asked.

"No more bread for us. We're on a diet."

The sense of this escaped me. I had heard of the Atkins Diet, but I didn't think the fare at the table was quite what the doctor had in mind. Four large men were sitting down to a pound of bacon, a large pack of sausages and a dozen and a half eggs, and they were on a diet.

"Yeah, we're stayin' away from the carbs. I've already lost five pounds."

I opened my mouth to protest, but decided my energies were better put to use having some of this opulent breakfast. As the five of us ate without further comment, I suddenly realized that our secretary wasn't with us.

"Where's Sharon?"

"She's off to the supermarket to pick up some steaks. We're having lunch here today."

The guys in my office all liked their work. They were good at what they did and often came in long before office hours started. A lot of their real work was out visiting farmers, but on days with weather as bad as this one, they would often stay in the office and finish up paperwork. When a group of food lovers like them (to be honest, I should say *us*) were all stuck inside for a day, usually someone suggested we all chip in a bit of cash for putting together a big feed. "You want to join us for lunch, Doc?"

"Sounds great. It looks slow today. I should be around for that." I fished through my wallet and brought out five dollars for my share.

Feeling a little bloated after two breakfasts, I was wondering about the wisdom of hobbit-eating habits when Sharon returned. The wind blew in through the door as she banged off her boots and carried two plastic bags to her desk.

"Some feed today," she told me. "I got steaks and a couple of pies. Dex brought in potatoes, Dwight has some smoked caplin, and Bryan has carrot and turnip. I made up a big salad last night."

Apparently this meal had been planned the afternoon before. I was feeling I hadn't contributed my share.

"How about if I peel some potatoes and carrots?" I offered.

In the class structure of our office, I knew that this would be the realistic limit of my allowed participation in the meal. The other guys could cook, and cook well. Early on in my work with them, I realized—we all realized—I wasn't in the same culinary league as them.

Sharon smiled, reached under her desk and handed me a bag of vegetables. The home of the provincial Department of Agriculture in Carbonear was one group of offices in a building that housed a number of other government groups. We all shared a large kitchen off the hall that ran between our suites.

As I sauntered down to the kitchen with my vegetables, it struck me—not for the first time—what a great group I worked with. No one ever seemed to argue about who was to do work around the office; it always got done. When non-work chores like peeling came up, there was never a fuss. No one ever complained about any of the meals that were prepared. Perhaps that was because they were without exception excellent and I never cooked.

I was through the potatoes and had about half of the carrots done when Sharon stuck her head into the kitchen. "Phone for you."

I returned to our office and the waiting phone.

"Hello?"

"That you, Doc?"

"It's me."

"Great day, Doc."

"It is. What's up?"

"I needs ya. It's me cow."

I recognized the voice and the unhelpful manner of presenting a problem. "Is this Tom?"

"Yeah. I needs ya."

"What's the trouble?"

"It's me cow."

"What's your cow's trouble?"

"She can't have her calf. She's been pushing since first thing this morning."

"Okay, Tom. I'll come up to your place right away."

"Better not."

"Why?"

"'Cause she's up in Bill's barn out by the incinerator."

I didn't want to get into why Tom's cow was in someone else's barn. There was a calf to deliver and a big dinner to be eaten. "I'll be right there."

Even though calvings were more fun than peeling potatoes, it disappointed me to leave the warmth of the kitchen. Even with coveralls and a heavy jacket on, a chill ran down my back as my dog and I went back out into the storm.

The snow hadn't yet been plowed on the road to the incinerator, so I would have to walk nearly a quarter of a mile to Bill's barn. Although it was uncomfortable rummaging through the back of the truck for equipment, I was careful to get everything I might possibly need for the work ahead. I had no intention of walking through the wind and snow any more than I had to. Mats sensibly decided he would wait this one out in the cab.

Just before I closed up the back of the truck, a piece of green rubber hiding far down in one compartment caught my eye. This was a calving suit that had been passed down to me from the last vet in the practice. I had never used it before because it looked cumbersome, but I wondered if it might be useful this time. The suit's purpose was to keep a vet relatively clean while doing a dirty job. This just might make me a little more presentable for the meal I was looking forward to.

With the calving equipment inside a bucket in one hand, a drug case in the other and the calving suit slung around my shoulders, I humped over to the barn. My rubber boots, which pulled on over regular shoes, weren't designed for the foot of snow on the path.

Bill was in the barn sitting on a bale of hay, and he started as though I had woken him up. The lack of tracks into the barn made me wonder how long he had been there.

"Is Tom around?"

"Nope. He's run down to the wharf to bring some grub down to the boat. We're headed out again tonight."

Tom and Bill worked fishing and spent long periods out on the sea when they weren't home with their cattle.

Bill rubbed his face and walked around to the back of one of the cows in the barn. "Here's the missus with the trouble. I've got some water boiled up for ya."

It seemed this was going to be a comfortable job. The kettle meant I would have warm water to wash up in, and my calving suit was going to keep me spotless.

As Bill mixed the boiling water with some water from the tap, I pulled on the calving suit. This wasn't so bad after all. I wondered why I had never used the suit before.

After cleaning my arm and the back end of the cow, I reached inside to see what was happening in this delivery. Within a foot of entering, I felt a solid mass blocking my way in through the reproductive tract. The calf was coming back end first, with its hind legs folded forward—a breech delivery.

A calf in this position usually meant a reasonably straight-forward birth. The trick was to push it forward and grab hold of the hind legs. Once the legs were tipped back, you had to be sure to haul the calf out before it started to breathe. As long as the legs weren't too hard to get, the job could be quick. Thoughts of eating steak among friends urged me on.

But when I placed the palm of my hand on the calf's rump, I felt hair. This was odd. Often at this point in the delivery, the calf is still inside the amniotic sac. Exposed hair meant that the sac had already ruptured.

I pushed gently on the calf, and the mother immediately grunted and pushed against me. Evidently I was going to have to put a little effort into moving this fellow forward. Planting my feet back another foot from the cow, I leaned in hard.

The cow was taken by surprise and the calf slipped forward into the uterus. As soon as the calf moved, the cow pushed hard. Suddenly I felt a disconcerting warmth envelope my arm and shoulder, quickly followed by the sensation of fluid running down the inside of my clothing. I looked down. Liquid was pouring over the rims of my boots.

Usually a cow has her "water break"—gallons of it—during delivery. In this case, the amniotic sac had broken while the calf was jammed tightly against the rim of its mother's pelvis, keeping all that fluid dammed up inside. Until I pushed.

The wet warmth actually felt quite pleasant—at first. Then I realized that (a) I was thoroughly soaked and (b) this liquid was going to cool off very quickly. Before continuing, I pulled off and emptied my boots. I sat on the floor draining, and put the boots back on.

The rest of the job wasn't too bad. The calf wasn't huge, and I could catch each of his thighs fairly easily. A second repositioning straightened the back legs. The calf slurped out with a gentle tug.

As the liquid chilled I was becoming more and more uncomfortable. Moving around was quickly becoming unpleasant.

With the calf out and his navel dipped in iodine, I wondered whether I should take the suit off. It was clammy and stuck to me like a bad dream, but taking it off would only leave me colder. I told Bill that I would mail Tom my bill. I wasn't staying in the barn any longer than I had to.

The walk back to the truck was miserable. The suit rubbed, and my socks began an unstoppable trip down to my toes. The most comfortable parts of me were those that were exposed to the howling wind.

At the truck I peeled off the calving suit and threw it in the back. Back in the cab, Mats indicated that he felt I smelled . . . very interesting. Because the truck had been running recently, it didn't take long for the cab to warm up. This thankfully took some of the chill out of me, but as the temperature in the truck rose, the odour from my soaked clothes increased.

Looking down at the clock on the dashboard, I saw that lunch at the office would be well under way. Choosing malodour over chill, I left the heat on full as I drove back to the office. By the time I got close, the air in the truck was enough to bring tears.

I drove on past the office, thinking how nice it would be to get these clothes off and warm up in the shower at home. A warmed-up steak a little later would suit me just fine.

27. My Biggest Patient

DR. JON LIEN TAUGHT animal behaviour at Memorial University and specialized in whales.

He was a wonderful and eccentric man. He was always excited about his work and full of new ideas. One time I passed him driving slowly along the road and I noticed that he had a book propped on the steering wheel and was reading as he drove. I honked the horn and pulled over for a chat. Jon explained that he was thinking about giving beekeeping a try and was reading up on it.

It was Jon who brought me together with my biggest-ever patient.

Before the moratorium in 1992, cod fishing was a major industry in Newfoundland. One of the popular fishing methods was with the cod trap: a series of net funnels leading to a net pen. One problem with cod traps was that whales swimming by a trap would sometimes catch their flukes or tails in some of the netting. Once caught, they would thrash about and wind more and more of the net around their bodies. Because whales are mammals that must breathe air, they drown if unable to surface.

Trapped whales presented a losing situation for everyone. The whales damaged or destroyed the traps and often perished in the process. Fishermen were furious when one of these monsters ruined the equipment that they relied on for their livelihood. The whales, while saying little about the situation, were no doubt just as displeased.

Jon put much of his efforts into eradicating this problem. He developed underwater warning systems that kept the whales away from nets and he worked with fishermen to help educate them about the value of the whales.

Jon also loved working in close proximity to these wonderful giants. Over the years he developed methods of freeing whales caught in fishing gear and taught his techniques to many fishermen.

I had met Jon when we both attended a lecture in St. John's. I let him know then that I was interested in helping out in any way that I could with his whale work. That was just the beginning of my adventures with Jon.

One summer afternoon, he called to let me know that a whale was caught in a trap very close to my house. He asked if I would like to go out on the water to help free the animal.

It took me no time to grab a set of rain clothes and drive over to the wharf in Carbonear. As I pulled up to the wharf, I could see Jon backing a trailer loaded with a Zodiac—an inflatable dinghy—down the slipway into the ocean. I walked down to the wharf to watch how this launching was going to be done. From experience, I knew that everything Jon did was done in a big, exuberant way.

The Zodiac was untied from the trailer, and on the wharf beside the slipway a man in a very new and expensive-looking set of rain clothes was holding a rope attached to the boat.

Jon yelled out "Hang on!" and furiously backed down the slipway. My first thought was that at this rate the truck and trailer would end up in the water along with the Zodiac.

Leaning precariously out the truck window, Jon jammed on the brakes the moment the top of the trailer went under the surface. The Zodiac made a spasmodic jerk and left the trailer just as Jon put the truck into drive and screeched up the ramp. It wasn't the prettiest launch I'd ever seen, but it certainly worked.

Jon parked the truck and ran over to where the well-dressed rope holder and I were standing.

"Great day, isn't it? This is going to be a special day."

Every day was a great day for Jon, but I could see from his enthusiastic eyes that something extraordinary was happening today.

"Bob, this is Andrew Peacock. He's the local vet and he comes out with me sometimes to help the whales. Andrew, this is Bob Johnston. He's with Sun Electronics in Texas. Bob has brought along a special electrocardiogram machine and we're going to see if we can do some heart monitoring on the humpback that's stuck in a net out there. No one has ever done this on a whale in the wild."

Jon had contacted the electronics corporation and convinced them that it would be great publicity for them if they gave him an EKG machine that would work on a whale. What better advertising than saying that your machine was able to work on the largest mammal on the planet? Jon felt that if he could successfully monitor a whale's heart, it would be one more way to assess the health of these mysterious animals when they were in trouble. It was no surprise to me that he had persuaded the company to send him their latest portable machine, housed in a waterproof case, and a digital audio tape recorder to document the monitoring.

As well as Bob, the company had sent two senior officials from Texas to watch the proceedings and operate the machines. I'm sure it was easy to find volunteers for this once-in-a-lifetime adventure. The fisherman who owned the trap that the whale was caught in agreed to take these two men out in his longliner. A 250-foot extension from the EKG lead kept them safely away from the action. Jon, Bob and I were to be up close to the whale and attach the EKG lead from the Zodiac.

After the local fisherman led us out to the site of his trap, the Zodiac stopped over the entrapped whale while the second boat waited a couple of hundred feet away. The two vessels were tethered by the EKG wires.

Most EKGs are done with three leads or more attached to particular parts of the body of the animal or person being monitored. This machine operated with a single lead that was to be attached to the animal with a large suction cup that looked something like the end of a toilet plunger.

Jon unzipped his bag and pulled out three diving masks and half a dozen knives of various shapes and lengths. He spat into his mask, rinsed it out, put it on and dunked his head over the side.

"There she is." His voice was nasal from the mask pinching off his nostrils.

He handed me a mask. "Have a look."

It's a bit of a shock sticking your head into the Atlantic at any time. This water never gets warm. The cold shock soon gave way to the realization that I was seeing something white under the boat. My first reaction was that the whale must be very deep to look that small. As I got my visual bearings underwater, I realized that the white object was only the whale's pectoral fin. I turned my head from one side to the other. There was grey whale skin as far as I could see in both directions. This animal had to be forty-five feet long.

I always thought that bulls were big animals. This changed everything. Bulls can weigh over a ton; humpback whales go up to forty-five tons. They can eat a bull's weight in minuscule plankton in one day. One of these behemoths was now sitting about ten feet under the small inflatable boat I was in.

"Get ready, she'll be up for air soon."

Though humpbacks can stay underwater for over half an hour, they usually come up for a breath every five to fifteen minutes. Breathing is done through the blowholes located on the top of the whale's head.

The water around our boat began to stir, and slowly the back of the whale came to the surface. We sat in awed silence as the blowholes came above the water and the whooshing sound of the blow began. Whales blowing are a sight and sound to stop the most jaded of us in our tracks. When a whale blows within ten feet of your small boat, you are not likely to ever forget the sensation. As well as the sound of the blow, I was amazed at the smell. This was a giant-sized case of bad breath.

Once we recovered from the awe of this display, we paddled the Zodiac a few feet in until we were actually touching the whale's back. Jon and I each took a knife, leaned far over the whale's back and cut any piece of net we could find. It was frantic work, as the whale stayed on the surface only for a few seconds.

The whale slowly drifted back into the depths.

Jon had done dozens of these whale rescues, but the thrill of the job had not diminished for him. "What a beauty!" he said. "She's got a lot of net on her. Did you see that rope wrapped around her tail? Next time up, we're getting the EKG lead on her." He checked his watch. "We have a bit of time now. I'd say she'll be back in five minutes or so. She knows we're here now, and I believe these animals know when you're trying to help them. But we've got to be care-ful—if she gets fed up with us, we'll have to back off."

"How can you tell when a whale's fed up?"

"If you see her flexing her tail, stop what you're doing and lie down in the boat. It's a bit like someone pulling their arm back to give you a swat."

Bob looked uncomfortable. "You're just kidding about that, Jon, aren't you?"

"No. Whales are safe to work around, but you've got to remember, they can flick a little boat like ours away like we would swat a fly."

Bob was looking a little green. I didn't think it was from the Zodiac bobbing up and down.

As Jon predicted, the whale surfaced in about five min-utes. With the EKG lead in his hand, Jon grabbed the rope that ran around the edges of the Zodiac and dunked his head and shoulders under the surface. For a second I was worried that he would flip over the side and we would soon be fishing him out of the water.

There was a splash as he surfaced and blew the water out of his mouth.

"Couldn't get the lead to stick on."

He inhaled deeply and plunged back over the side. With more surface commotion, he came back up, climbed aboard and ripped off his mask. "It's on. Let's get some more net cut off."

Jon stood up, and as he did so he kicked one of the knives into the side of the Zodiac. I heard a disturbing pop and a loud hiss as the section of the Zodiac facing the whale softened. Without much evidence of great concern, Jon pulled the knife out of the side and started slicing netting. I followed his lead, but as I cut I couldn't help noticing our boat's shrinking dimensions.

As before, the whale slipped below the surface after we had cut a little more of the netting away.

"Um, Jon, did you see the hole in our boat?"

"Oh, that's nothing. These Zodiacs have three chambers and they'll still float even with all three deflated."

"Do you believe that?"

"Probably not."

Bob was looking terror-stricken. "You're both crazy!" He stood up in our somewhat diminished vessel and started waving his arms wildly at the men in the fishing boat. The skipper of the longliner recognized his distress and drew his boat closer.

"Get me off this boat!" Bob yelled. "They're crazy!"

The longliner came alongside our stricken Zodiac, and Bob scrambled up the sides and over the gunwales. As they pulled away from us, Jon and I listened to a gradually fading tirade on the states of our collective sanity, the size of the whale and the general discomfort offered by the ocean.

"Guess he didn't like that hole in the boat. Okay, here she comes again."

This time when the whale surfaced, it was easier to lean over to cut the ropes, because we didn't have a raised side of the boat facing the whale. I think the suggestions that we were deranged pushed us to lean farther and cut more boldly to free the whale. It was as though we were proving there was some value to this strange adventure we were on.

After two more surfacings, we had cut away enough rope and netting that the whale was no longer tied down. As she submerged the last time there was a definite change. Instead of falling down into the water with her body level, she tipped her head down and moved with an obvious purpose. The EKG lead pulled free as she swam away. The last we saw was the characteristic flip of her tail above the surface.

We worried that we hadn't removed all of the rope from around the base of her tail and we would never know if this last bit of debris would be a problem. Perhaps it would entangle her again somewhere deep in the ocean, or perhaps it would work its way free.

With a measured sense of success and new hope for my largest patient, we started the engine and headed back to the wharf in our wounded Zodiac.

28. The Bribe

VISITS TO MAURICE'S PLACE were always interesting. He lived in Upper Island Cove, a community about half an hour away from my home. Linguistically and culturally, it might as well have been halfway around the world.

Upper Island Cove is a small town that in every way is just off the main road. The community sits perched on rock completely exposed to the North Atlantic. There isn't much shelter in the way of deep coves or covering vegetation. The wind blows through Upper Island Cove unimpeded.

It is the people, however, that make this community truly unique. They speak a dialect that is purely their own. Historians tell us that much of the population originated from Devon in England, but it is unlikely that anyone in Devon ever spoke the way that Island Covers do. When we first moved to Newfoundland, Ingrid would ask nurses to translate for her when people from the town came to see her in the emergency department.

The people of Upper Island Cove are noted for their music and humour. It seems that everyone there can play an instrument, and they all have a wonderful if somewhat strange sense of humour. Island Covers revel in their distinctiveness. While they aren't averse to feuds, they share a fierce loyalty to their community. It was common to hear dissertations from locals on the high intelligence and long list of achievements of natives of Island Cove.

Maurice epitomized everything about the community that was different. He was a short man with a luxuriant moustache and an ego that couldn't be levelled with a stick. He talked nonstop, and most of his talk centred on how amazing he was.

As I pulled into Maurice's driveway, I saw him resplendent in a garish purple tracksuit, framed in the open doorway of his garage. The garage was neat beyond reason. Three large freezers hinted at the volume of fish and game that he had squirrelled away. I didn't spend much time wondering where these bounties of the earth and sea had come from and how they came to be in his freezers. He was standing beside a high-end bag of hockey equipment and was rotating tape onto a stick.

Maurice started as soon as I opened the truck door.

"'Ow are ya today, my son? Look 'ere, this is some 'ocky stick. Do you play? No? Well, if ya did ya should 'ave a stick like this."

I broke in when he stopped to catch his breath. "Yeah, I play a bit of hockey, Maurice. Now, you've got some problems with your goats?"

"Yes, my son. Now them goats I 'ave is some cleva goats. There's nobody that 'as goats quite like 'em. I got 'em from a fella out in Bonne Bay. I was out there doin' a bit of business, if ya know what I mean."

I had no idea what he meant.

"Yes, I sees this feller out in a field with these lovely goats and I 'offas 'im a freezer I 'ave in the back for the three of 'em. He didn't see me comin', my son. They're lovely goats."

"Well, I guess we should get out and see them."

"Right on, right on, just let me finish putting this tape on . . . there. Did ya ever see a stick taped quite so neat as that? My son, there's a trick to this."

Maurice put down the tape and carefully placed the stick on a rack on the garage wall alongside three other weapons of sport. He put the equipment bag in its spot under the sticks and fluffed the sides out until it looked like an illustration in a catalogue. With this done, he turned, went to the door connecting the garage to the house and disappeared inside.

After a few minutes, he returned to the garage wearing a shining new set of coveralls and spotless boots. The coveralls said "Government of Newfoundland and Labrador" on the shoulders. I didn't remember that Maurice had worked for the government.

"Now these are the real fit out. 'Ave you got a pair like this?"

I had worked for the government for over a decade, but no, I didn't have a pair of coveralls as opulent as the ones he sported.

"You ready to see the goats, my son? They aren't heatin' to my satisfaction."

I had been ready since arriving, but there was nothing to gain by pointing this out.

As we walked to his barn, Maurice sang a song about a shipwreck and the beautiful maidens involved in the wreck. There didn't seem to be an off switch on the man.

The barn, like everything else around Maurice, was made

of only the best material. It looked more like a cottage than a place to house animals. The sides were covered with clapboard and painted yellow, the roof was shingled, and the small window wouldn't look out of place in a house.

Inside, it struck me right away that perhaps this barn was a little too well built. The air was stifling; the six goats and four sheep inside were too much for the little ventilation provided. There was a slight touch of ammonia in the atmosphere, and the coughing of the goats hinted at what was amiss.

"Looks like some of your animals have a bit of a coughing problem, Maurice."

"You're spot on, buddy. That is what their trouble is. Funny they would 'ave such a problem in a lovely barn like this."

"It's important that you provide fresh air for the animals. They need good fresh air to keep them healthy."

"Right on, right on. You're spot on with that, buddy. Now some other fellas round here don't worry 'bout stuff like that, but I always say you needs good fresh hair."

"Well, the way to get fresh air is to make sure the barn is well ventilated. To do that you need to have some way for the air to get in."

"Spot on, spot on—"

I cut him off before he could get wound up. "And in order to get the air in, you'll need to keep the doors and windows open."

"Spot on, buddy. I keep things open here all the time so they gets fresh hair. Now other guys with goats . . ."

I let him ramble awhile as I looked at the closed window and remembered how we had opened the barn door to get in.

"If I was you," I interrupted, "as well as keeping everything open, I'd get a drill and put some holes up through the soffits."

"Spot on, spot on." Maurice ground his cigarette out with his fingers, put it into his pocket and walked out of the barn.

I now had a quiet moment in which to examine the animals. None of them had a temperature, but when I checked them with my stethoscope, a few of them had too much noise in their lungs.

I had just finished looking over the last goat when I heard a whirring and grinding noise coming through the sides of the barn. Outside, Maurice had a new cigarette dangling from his lips and was drilling holes into the soffit with a cordless drill. Maurice wasn't one to procrastinate.

"Looks good, Maurice."

"Right on, buddy. I thought it might be a good idea to put some 'oles into the soffit to ventilate the fresh hair."

I stopped myself from saying "spot on."

"I think improving the air in your barn will be all that you'll need to do, but just to be on the safe side, I'll get you a bit of antibiotic for a couple of the goats and one sheep that are a bit worse than the rest."

As I went back to the truck for the drugs, I could hear Maurice starting into another tune. He had finished drilling the soffit by the time I returned to the barn and I had to wait for him to take the drill back to the house. I had no doubt that it was put away neatly.

I was not surprised that Maurice knew how to inject the drugs into the animals. His method was just a little superior to that of the other farmers in the area, and he agreed heartily with my suggestions on how often the shots should be given and how long the treatment should continue. By the time I reviewed the treatment regimen, he was talking as though the whole procedure had been his idea.

As we left the barn, Maurice stopped and closed the door. I suppose it made the barn neat.

"Maurice," I said, "remember the fresh air."

"Right on, right on." He turned back, opened the door and fastened it with a piece of twine from inside the barn.

As he busied himself in the garage, I retrieved my receipt book from the truck. "That'll be fifty bucks, tax and all," I said as I started to write.

Maurice reached into his pocket and pulled out a twenty-dollar bill. "Doc, why don't you just put this in your small pocket and forget you were 'ere."

This was a new approach for me. I hadn't run into a blatant bribe in my practice before. There was something about Maurice that I liked, though, and I felt I should explain in a way he would understand. A discussion of morality and decency probably wouldn't go anywhere.

"See, Maurice, the thing is, if I don't write up bills and send money in to the government, they'll think I'm not doing any work. If that happens, I won't have a job and you won't have a vet."

"Right on, right on." He pulled out another thirty dollars and handed the full amount to me.

As I finished the bill, he sauntered over to one of the freezers and dipped inside. I was just quick enough to catch a frozen package of cod that he threw across the garage.

"Now, my son, you won't find better fish than that. Fry some of that hup when you get 'ome. I guarantee you it'll be the best you've ever 'ad.

It seemed there were no hard feelings. I left with some cod and a grin as Maurice started into another song.

29. Moose Rides Shotgun

DEALING WITH WILD ANIMALS is not like dealing with domestic ones. We don't know much about them and they don't know much about us.

Wild animals generally don't like being seen by people. They will do anything they can to stay away from us. It causes them great stress to be penned up or to be touched.

Often our first, well-meaning responses are more harmful than helpful. Every year people try to rescue young wild animals that seem to be alone by capturing them and bringing them in to wildlife officials.

Many of these "orphans" would have been fine if left alone. A moose calf found by itself may be only temporarily separated from its mother. It is even possible that the mother is hiding nearby to avoid being seen by the calf's "rescuers."

Sometimes, of course, wild animals are true orphans, abandoned too young and in real danger. In situations like this, rescue can be of real value. It takes careful observation and patience to determine whether any young animal is a true orphan.

In early fall one year, a group of hunters found an impressive female moose drinking from the waters of Swansea pond, just outside of the town of Victoria. With a single shot the animal was brought down. Only when the group came up to claim their prey did they notice that a very young calf was standing nearby.

Later that afternoon, one of the hunters phoned me and asked what should be done about the abandoned youngster. I got in touch with the local conservation officer, and we drove down to the pond and spent two fruitless hours scouting the area for signs of the little moose.

The next morning I heard from a man who had been out fishing at Swansea pond. He reported that he had seen a very small moose calf. I had a number of calls scheduled for the day, so I wasn't able to get back to my office until early evening. Sharon told me that Tom Antle from Victoria wanted me to phone him.

I dialed the number. "Hi, is Tom around?"

"He's not here right now." It was an older, quavering voice. I assumed that I had reached Tom's mother.

"This is the vet calling. Tom called me."

"Oh hello, Doctor, how are you today?"

"I'm fine, thank you. Do you know what Tom called me for?"

"It's a lovely day, Doctor, the sun was certainly something today, wasn't it?"

"It certainly was a lovely day, Mrs. Antle. Do you know where Tom is?"

"Tom?"

"Yes, Tom."

"I'm not sure what Tom called you for, he's out in the barn with that cute little moose, my, what a darlin' she is."

"Thanks, Mrs. Antle. I think I'll just run down to your place right now."

I had a pretty good idea why Tom had called me and I didn't think that I was going to get much more information from his mother. I did know that whatever happened at the farm, there would be a cup of tea and cookies waiting that could not be refused.

Mats and I drove up to the farm and found Tom standing out in his drive. Tom was shaped like a strip of wire. He was quiet and always polite, but he had a reputation for being a hard man when he drank. A local story had it that Tom had been ejected from a drinking establishment one night. He found his way back in through a new door he added that very night with a chainsaw. Apparently nothing was ever said to the police, and he spent the next two days repairing the building.

"Hello, Doctor. I suppose you've come to see me moose?"

"I have. And how did you end up with a moose, Tom?"

"Me'n Mudder were out for a run on the quad around noon and I seen the little bugger standin' there by the pond up the road. Poor thing looked lost so I shuffed Mudder on home out of it and caught holt of 'im. He got a ride here on the back where Mudder usually sits."

Tom's mother looked to be around eighty, and I couldn't imagine him making her walk back the three or four miles from the pond to his house.

"So did you go back for your mother after you brought the moose home?"

"My son, Mudder's right tough. Besides, I was busy watchin' the little bugger once I got home."

"Let's have a look at him."

Tom led me into his barn. All his cattle were out on the community pasture for the summer. It took a few seconds for my eyes to adjust to the darkness and bring the sole resident into view. In the far corner, a very small moose calf was lying in a pile of feed bags. As we entered, it let out a pathetic little mewl that could only be described as lonely.

Part of me was frustrated at Tom's interference in the life of this poor creature, but on the whole he'd done the right thing. This had to be the same calf that had lost its mother the previous day, and without Tom's intervention it might have starved alone.

"What were you planning on doing with the moose, Tom?"

"I figgered I'd keep her a few days and then call Wildlife."

"Well, Tom, it's great that you picked up the calf. But you know, she really needs to be somewhere that she can be looked after properly."

"I sove her, all right. The little bugger woulda perished if Mudder'n me hadn't come along. But I suppose you're right. I guess I better call Wildlife."

"Tell you what, Tom. You just keep her here in the barn tonight. I know you'll look after her well. I'll call the Wildlife guys and get her taken to the Salmonier Nature Park tomorrow morning."

When I got home, I called the local conservation officer and let him know that I had found the moose calf we had been looking for the night before. He was pleased to hear the calf was doing well, but said that he was leaving early the next morning for a caribou project on the other end of the island. It wouldn't be possible for him to take the calf to the nature park.

My truck wasn't built for transporting animals. It was a three-quarter-ton four-wheel-drive pickup with a fibreglass body dropped into the box. The box was a great help for vet work. There was hot and cold running water—when the electrical system worked—and locking compartments all around to hold drugs and equipment. None of the spaces were big enough, though, to hold a baby moose.

I reasoned that the moose really should get to the park in the morning. Just because my truck wasn't designed as a small moose carrier, I wasn't going to miss the opportunity to go for a drive with this fascinating animal and help bring it to a new, safe home.

In the morning I drove out to Tom's again to pick up the moose. Tom's mother was out in the garden in front of the barn expressing the conflicting emotions of what a cute little animal the moose was and what a fine bit of stew she'd make someday. Tom was off fishing for the morning, so I didn't have any help moving the moose. After a couple of sprints across the barn, she fortunately came around to the conclusion that it wouldn't be too bad to be held by a strange person.

I cornered the moose, and after putting my arms around her chest and behind her rump, managed to fold her legs in underneath her body. I was surprised how easy to carry she was. She couldn't have weighed more than forty pounds.

The only place that the moose would fit in the truck was the footwell of the passenger's side of the cab. With her legs tucked well under her body, she fit well and didn't seem overly stressed. I wondered whether she even felt a little more secure in this dark, enclosed shelter.

After convincing Mrs. Antle that I really couldn't stop in for another bit of tea and some toast, I was off with my moose. The drive started well, and it looked like the moose transportation was going to be a breeze. Usually, I drove with Mats as co-pilot and CBC for entertainment. This trip was to be a little more spartan. I wasn't certain that the dog and moose would be good companions for the hour it took to get to the park, so Mats had a day off. The radio was always helpful, but I wasn't sure the moose would share my enthusiasm for daytime public radio programming.

As I hit the highway I glanced down at the dash. With a start, I realized I didn't have enough gas to get all the way to the park. In the excitement of leaving to pick up my passenger, I had completely forgotten to check the fuel level.

I drove for half an hour before I found somewhere to pull in at Clarke's Beach for some gas. The moose had been relaxed so far, and all I needed was a little co-operation while I pumped and paid. I gently slowed coming into the gas station. The calf never stirred as I cautiously opened and closed my door as quietly as I could manage. As I opened the gas cap and inserted the nozzle, I watched the passenger side of the cab for signs of moose distress. There were none. With great relief I replaced the cap and sprinted for the cash register.

There was no lineup and payment was mercifully fast. I slipped the receipt into my pocket and headed out the door. Immediately, I could see that the calf had stood up in the footwell and was peering out the side window. And a heavy little man who had pulled in behind me was staring back at him. I dashed for the truck.

"Some weird-lookin' dog you got there, buddy."

I grunted something that I hoped sounded half-friendly and jumped into the truck. The calf was startled by my sudden reappearance in the enclosed area and scrambled up onto the seat. There wasn't enough height for her to stand, and her cramped position upset her further. She thrashed against the window.

I slid across the seat and wrapped my arms around her body. Without control of her legs she got a few slashes in before I had her properly restrained. It took considerable contortions to fold her back into a package that would fit in front of the seat.

The heavy man was now peering in the passenger window through tunnelled hands. He shook his head in disbelief and his lips moved. It was impossible to hear his comments with the ruckus in the truck, and I really wasn't much interested in a conversation at this point anyway.

With the calf under tenuous control, I started the truck and drove to a more solitary part of the service station parking lot. The moose and I had steamed up the cab, so I rolled down my window for a little fresh air. In the rear-view mirror I could see my spectator approaching across the lot.

"Hey, buddy!"

This was no time for an address on the wonders of wildlife and their transportation, so I quickly pulled out onto the highway. However, my passenger was no longer satisfied to sit quietly on the floor. She had seen the glorious vistas offered by the window and at the very least wanted another look. For the rest of the drive to the park, I kept one hand on the steering wheel and used the other to periodically push the moose's head down. By the time I got to the Salmonier I was ready for a rest.

We moved the calf into a small pen that was away from the public viewing area. Staff started feeding her with a baby bottle.

Raising orphan moose is notoriously difficult, but the park staff had an excellent record of success. In the days before I was associated with them, they kept a lactating goat on site that uncomplainingly suckled successive orphan moose. By the time I worked at the park, they had settled for bottle feeding.

Wild animals cannot be safely returned to the wild after they have been hand-raised. Because they learn to trust people, they would be as trusting of hunters as they were of their surrogate parents. This moose calf would have naturally died shortly after her mother was shot, but instead, she lived a long life in the relative comfort of the park.

30. He or She?

MONDAY MORNING BEGAN with what sounded like a routine call.

"Can you come up and see Gerald Durdle's cow?"

"I can be up there this morning if you give me directions. Is this Mrs. Durdle?"

"Oh, I'm not Mrs. Durdle, my darling. Gerald's woman is in the hospital. She has bad nerves, you know—tried to do herself in one time last winter. Poor Gerald with the wife in the hospital and him with his bad foot, sometimes I wonder how the poor man manages at all."

When I sensed her stopping for a breath I cut in. "Do you know what's wrong with Gerald's cow?"

"Well now, Doctor, it's like this. I've never seen Gerald's cow, and to be truthful with you, I don't care if I ever do. He's over in that house by himself with all those cats and I don't know how he looks after himself. Now back when his woman was better, she used to be a wonderful cook, she made the best flipper pie of anyone on this shore."

With another pause I leapt in again. "Could you tell me how to find Gerald?"

"Yes, my ducky, I could do that. Do you know where Island Cove is? Well if you don't, I guess you won't be much help to Gerald. Anyway, as you come along through Island Cove, you'll come across Clifford Snelgrove's store. Now just a gunshot past that there's a road turns off and Gerald lives on that road, you can't miss him. Don't mind the cats when you go to Gerald's. I suppose they're all he has now. It's shockin' how nobody ever goes over to visit that man. If I had more time I'd—"

"Excuse me, ma'am, but I have a couple of people waiting here to see me and I have to get running."

After selling two bottles of sheep wormer and reassuring a worried horse owner that it was perfectly normal for her mare to go a day over eleven months in her pregnancy, I was ready for the road.

The trip to Lower Island Cove is a pleasant thirty-minute drive along a winding road that never strays too far from the ocean. On the stretch by Kingston the road swings out close to a hundred-foot drop to the sea, affording an unobstructed panorama of Conception Bay, with rocky islands pushing up out of the water to the south.

I remembered Clifford Snelgrove's store from many previous journeys along the north shore, but my directions beyond this were far from precise. Apparently Gerald lived on a road about a gunshot from the store, but I hadn't been told if the road was to the left or the right. From years of taking directions over the phone, I had a pretty good idea what a gunshot meant. This could be a distance anywhere from about fifty yards to over a mile.

It turned out that three roads fit my directions for finding Gerald's. I decided to take the first road to the left and see if

I could find someone to give me more exact instructions. About a mile in, I spotted a short, round man with an exceptional white beard leaning on a woodpile smoking a cigarette. I guessed that he was getting ready to cut up some wood into pieces that would fit into his stove. Or perhaps he was just leaning on the woodpile and smoking.

I rolled down my window. "Morning. Can you tell me where Gerald Durdle lives?"

"Ge-rald," he drawled. It wasn't a question or an answer; it seemed more like a meditation on the sound of the name. "You mean Gerald Durdle?"

"Yes, Gerald Durdle. He's got cows."

"Well, Gerald lives on this road."

"Could you tell me which house is his?"

"Yes sir. He lives in a white bungalow, set back a nice piece from the road."

This wasn't much help, as three-quarters of the houses I had passed were white, and "a nice piece" was a unit of distance that made "a gunshot" look precise. I tried a different approach.

"How far in the road is he?"

"Let me see now . . . well, he would be the"—he looked up into the sky for the answer—"first house in."

"Thanks, skipper."

These weren't the best instructions that I'd ever been given, but they definitely weren't the worst.

Gerald's house was a dilapidated white bungalow that looked as though it had been built in the 1950s. Even with its peeling paint, it exuded more character than the well-manicured plastic bungalows farther in the road. The house was surrounded by weather-beaten pines, and two barrels planted with small dead trees sat in front of it.

I knocked on the door, then pulled it open and leaned my head into the porch. "Hello! Gerald. Anybody home?"

"Come in. Come in, boy. I'll just be a minute."

I stepped inside.

My first impression was of cat urine. The stinging sensation of ammonia assaulted my nose and eyes. It was hard to imagine how anyone could be comfortable in such an atmosphere.

The dead trees outside and the heavy cat smell prepared me for a mess inside. Yet I was pleasantly surprised by the neat and cozy kitchen that led off from the porch. The black-and-white tiles on the floor had been recently washed, the table by the window was uncluttered, and the rocking chair in the corner was neatly covered with a colourful afghan.

Gerald limped into the kitchen. He used every chair and solid object he could find along his way to help him walk. His face contorted every time his left foot touched the ground.

I recognized Gerald. I had seen him a few times before in our office, when he had come in to pick up supplies for his cattle. He was a short and slightly overweight man in his sixties with a friendly round face. Now, his grin flashed to a grimace as he lowered himself into the rocking chair and just as quickly returned to a grin as he settled in.

"It's good to see you, Doc. My bull's not very good, you see. I wonder if you could take a look at her for me."

"Sure, Gerald, that's what I'm here for. Where's your bull?"

"She's out on the Low Point pasture."

"Is she in a pen out there?" If Gerald was going to call his bull a she, I supposed I might as well join in.

"No, boy, she's out with the other cows."

This was going to be interesting. I was supposed to examine an animal that had been running loose with sixty other animals over hundreds of acres of pasture. We would be lucky if we could *find* the bull, and it would take a number of fleet-footed helpers to even move the animal into someplace where I could examine him. Her.

"Is there anyone who can help us round up the bull?"

"Tom Osbourne's son said he was going to drop over this morning, but he got called in to the fish plant last night and he'll still be in bed. There's nobody else about. But you and I shouldn't have any trouble getting that bull."

This wasn't looking very promising. "How's your foot, Gerald?"

"Boy, it's not very good. I fell down the steps last week and I must have done something to it. I didn't get to sleep at all last night, it was such a wonderful bad pain. At least the swelling has gone down enough that I can get on me boots now." Gerald bent down and took off his slippers. His lower leg was grossly swollen, and an angry red colour showed above the top of his sock.

"Have you seen a doctor about that, Gerald? It doesn't look very good."

"No, boy. The last time I hurt this leg, the doctor made me put a cast on it. That cast was the worst thing I ever suffered. There's no way nobody is going to put a cast on me again."

He carefully shifted his body in the chair and managed to pull on his right boot without putting any pressure down on his left foot. He took a deep breath and pulled the remaining boot onto the swollen left foot—though not without grimacing and biting on his lower lip.

"Are you sure you're okay, Gerald?"

"Just give me a minute and I'll be fine." He stared straight ahead and took three long and deep breaths. Then he pushed himself to his feet, grabbed hold of the edge of the table and grinned. "There, see? I'm perfect."

He looked a long way from perfect to me, but faced with his resolve in getting his boots on and his faith that the two of us could catch the bull, I scarcely wanted to keep him from our adventure.

"Give me your arm there, Gerald, and I'll help you out to the truck."

"Thanks, Doc, but I'm fine."

Gerald made his way through the kitchen with the help of any horizontal surface that presented itself, pausing only to lift a salt-and-pepper cap from the kitchen counter and pull it on. Going down the three front steps was an effort, but he did make it to my truck. I pushed ahead and opened the passenger door. Gerald half jumped and crawled his way up onto the seat, breathing heavily.

Mats had been sitting on the driver's seat while I was in talking to Gerald. I'm sure that dogs think of the driver's seat as the top dog's place and so take it over at any opportunity. Now, as I walked around to my side of the truck, I could hear Gerald talking to Mats.

"Hello, doggie. How are you? I bet you'd like to meet my cats."

Mats was too busy sniffing this man who smelled like a cat to pay any attention to anything he was saying. After a few quick runs up and down Gerald's near leg with his nose, Mats decided that this guy was all right. As I stepped up into my seat, Mats slipped over onto Gerald's lap.

"Oh, you're a friendly doggie. Do you want me to rub your ears?"

Mats licked his lips and closed his eyes as he luxuriated in the attention.

We drove up to the pasture, where we found another unexpected impediment.

"Oh no," I said. "They've locked us out." The gate on the short lane leading to the pasture was locked with a chain; there was no easy way in to the fence that surrounded the pasture. It would be difficult enough for Gerald to get over the uneven ground of the pasture, but this fence was surely impassable.

"I can get over that thing, boy."

I cringed as Gerald hobbled up to the fence, gripped the fence post and lifted his good foot up onto a strand of wire. With a mighty effort he pushed off the top of the post, balanced precariously over the top of the fence and came down hard on the other side.

"Boy, that hurt," he said. It had to be an understatement.

We rested for a moment while Gerald regained his composure, then set off for the pasture gate, forty yards away. Thanks to the flat ground, no doubt, Gerald's walking seemed to improve.

Our next disappointment came at the gate to the pasture field: the nearest animals we could see were easily a gunshot away. (This would be one of those long gunshots.)

"I don't see me bull in with those ones up there. That brown one might be her, but I don't think so." He gestured at the crowd of about fifty cattle, most of which were some shade of brown.

"That's too bad, Gerald. I guess we won't get a chance to look at your bull today, unless we can find someone else to give us a hand catching her."

He ignored me, leaned over the edge of the fence and put his hands up to his mouth. "Come cow, come cow, come cow!"

Almost immediately a few of the nearest animals lifted their heads from eating and looked our way. After a moment's hesitation, a few started ambling toward us. The migration gained momentum as more and more started moving, and before long most were galloping in our direction.

Gerald's eyes sparkled and a smile came to his face. "There she is. She lost some weight since she came here in the spring."

As the cattle came nearer, I had a chance to get a closer look at Gerald's bull. He looked bright and moved well, but his ribs were prominent and his coat had an unhealthy dullness.

I figured this was going to be as much of an examination of my patient as I was going to get. Without further inspection, the obvious problems were likely worms and bullying. Many of the local pastures did not have a consistent deworming policy, and even clean animals brought in during the spring could be full of them by fall. Another problem I saw quite often on these pastures was submissive animals that were pushed out of the way so much by the other cattle that they didn't get the opportunity to eat well.

I told Gerald, "I'm going to get something to pour onto her back in case she's full of worms. The other thing I would suggest is to get some buddies to help you get her onto a truck and feed her up at home for a while."

I jogged back to the truck and picked up a bottle of pour-on anti-parasite drug. Pouring the dewormer over the bull's back was not as easy as I thought it would be. As nonchalantly as I walked among the cattle, the bull seemed to always sense that I had targeted him. He slipped around animals that were between him and me and generally made it difficult for me to get near him. Eventually, after three near passes, I got close enough to pour the drug over his back.

The fence Gerald and I had stood at met a second fence that divided off a confinement area with a small, gated opening. I wondered if it would be possible to direct Gerald's bull into this smaller area with a few other animals. If I could do that, and then simply chase the other animals back out, I would be able to make a more complete examination of the bull.

I opened the gate and patiently walked back and forth through the cattle. My plan was to persuade a number of them to move toward the opening in the hope some would decide to go through. This kind of animal-driving usually takes more than one person, but it was worth a try. Luck was with me, as Gerald's bull wandered over toward the open gate and without as much as a gesture from me decided to walk through. I ran up, closed the gate and smiled.

It was easy from this vantage to chase him into the catching corral and down through a narrow alley into the head gates. With the bull's head caught in the gates, I was able to examine him thoroughly and safely. I took his temperature, listened to his heart and lungs, looked through his hair for bugs and had a good look into his mouth. The only information I gleaned beyond what I had expected was a further complication to Gerald's animal's gender. She was a he, of course, but not quite a bull. The animal had been incompletely castrated and so was actually something between a bull and a steer. I soon clarified his identity with a scalpel.

After I released the steer from the head gate, I suggested to Gerald that he leave him—her—in the confinement area for the time being. There was plenty of grass in this area and no other animals to harass him while he waited to be taken home.

The trip back had to be as difficult as getting there, but Gerald appeared more at ease. He climbed over the fence quicker and didn't even pause between the fence and the truck.

After we said our goodbyes in front of his house, I watched for a moment to make sure that he navigated his way in through his front door safely. He took two steps at a time on his way up to the porch.

31. One Tough Pig

DARYA, A COLLEAGUE FROM the Corner Brook office, had been visiting with the St. John's vets for a few days, studying their new ultrasound equipment. She arranged to spend a day with me before heading home.

The day began with a horse castration. This was worth seeing, because I used a different technique from hers. We discussed the pros and cons as we drove between calls.

The second call was another castration in Dildo, Gord's pig this time. The sun was shining as we turned into the farm. Gord lived right on the bay, and the day's warmth and the glittering water set the scene for a pleasant afternoon of work.

Gord was a large, well-muscled man with an impressive white moustache. He had just retired from maintenance work on the DEW Line in the Far North. His military shirt with torn-off sleeves added to the impression that this was not a man to be messed with. Every time I saw him he was busy; with Gord, there was always more work than there was time.

As Darya and I got out of the truck, we heard a banging noise up the hill from us. After a short walk, we found Gord driving fence posts into the ground with an enormous sledge-hammer. When he saw us, he pulled a handkerchief from his pocket and wiped it over his severe grey crewcut.

"You got a girl with ya! That's pretty good."

"Hi, Gord. This is Darya. She's a vet from Corner Brook."

"A girl *and* a vet, that's even better. I guess I don't need to help you with that pig. I'm damn busy here with this fence. It's the pig by itself in the last pen up in the barn."

"No problem, we'll go and do that up."

Darya and I crossed the short field to Gord's barn. The barn was unusual even by rural Newfoundland standards. The roof was rounded and supported by beams that looked to me to be at least four times as big as they needed to be for the size of the barn. The main floor was similarly over-engineered, with thick planks and giant beams.

The inside of the barn, though, smelled just the same as most pig barns. If you are used to pigs, the pungent odour is perhaps even pleasant. But it's not for everyone. The concentration of withering funk in pig barns depends on how well ventilated the building is. For all the extravagance in the construction of this barn, its ventilation was lacking.

Darya and I walked down the cement walkway. Every phase of the pigs' growth took place in this one room. First, we saw sows in crates with their newborn piglets fighting over the best spots for a drop of milk. Next were pens with young growing pigs. These animals always fascinated me with their obvious curiosity about everything that went on around them. When we had entered the barn they were all sleeping, lying across each other with no cares in the world. Our first steps through the door woke one pig, and his disturbed snorts brought the rest to life. In no time, all of them were standing at the edge of their pen trying to get a look at or a smell of the new visitors.

In the last pen we found our patient. While the crates containing the sows and the pens with the young pigs were quite clean, his was filled with over a foot of sloppy manure.

Pigs are usually castrated when very young. This makes them much easier to handle and results in less stress for both the castrator and the castratee. But this was no young pig. Facing us down across the bars of his cage was a four-hundred-pound boar.

This was going to be interesting. I had castrated a boar larger than this when I was a student, but I wasn't really satisfied with the procedure we'd used. Young piglets could be castrated with little anaesthesia of any kind. This one would require a different approach.

I headed back to the truck to pick up some material while Darya hiked back up to Gord's fence to make absolutely sure that this big boar was to be castrated. Castration of mature boars is rare, one reason being that the meat of a pig that has matured intact will often have a very strong smell.

Gord confirmed that the adult boar was indeed the castratee, and so I laid out my drugs and surgical kit. I had also brought along my pig snare. Unlike the snare used for deliveries, this is an instrument of restraint, consisting of a three-foot metal handle with a cable noose at one end. You tighten the noose over the top jaw of a pig to cause enough distraction that minor work can be done with relative ease.

We looked at our equipment and the pig. Every time we sized him up he seemed a little larger. We agreed that some kind of sedation would be easier on both us and the pig. The problem was that we needed a drug that was both safe for the animal and whoever eventually ate the meat. Most of the best sedatives were not registered for use in animals intended for the table.

We finally decided that we should try a drug called Stresnil, which is used mainly for pigs that are being transported. It calms them down and keeps them from fighting.

Our plan was for Darya to distract the pig from the front of the pen while I leaned in over the side to inject the drug. The pig was plenty interested in Darya when she stood in front of him, but he had no intention of letting me reach any part of his body from outside the pen. Our ruse clearly wasn't going to work.

We decided to refine our tactic a little by having Darya hold out a bucket of pig feed to further distract our intended victim. The feed got his full attention. He snorted and groaned with great pleasure as he drove his head into the pail.

More boldness was required. It occurred to me that while the pig was so engrossed in the feed I could slip over the fence undetected and silently administer the sedative.

Darya returned to her post at the front of the pig and offered the pail. He glanced at me out of the corner of his eye before diving in again.

I gave him a few moments to really get into the feast before I carefully lowered myself over the fence. Manure sucked my boots in place. When I lifted a foot, it made a sound like a suction cup pulled off glass. The boar let out a ferocious snort and stopped eating. I held my ground, hoping his revelry in the pail would restart. But the pig jerked his head up, knocking the pail out of Darya's hands and spilling feed around the pen. He pivoted toward me faster than an animal with four legs should have been able to. He squealed again, dropped his head and charged. Demonstrating the advantages of having two legs, I turned even faster than the pig and lunged for the fence. I caught the top rail with my hand and vaulted to safety.

Despite my obvious display of cowardice and poor judgment, I felt some consolation that I had made it over the fence. I was also relieved that my boots had worked free from the manure so quickly and followed me to safety.

Darya pointed at the spot where I had been standing. "Look! Your thermometer."

In the course of my rapid retreat, my thermometer had fallen out of the breast pocket of my coveralls.

"We'll get that back eventually, and if he does step on it, it's not a big loss."

But the pig had other plans. After threatening us with three charges at the edge of the pen, he turned his attention to this shining glass tube. Without hesitation, he took it into his mouth. With a loud crunch, he pulverized the thermometer between his molars.

Darya and I looked at each other.

"Mercury can't be very good for a pig," I said. "Have you ever heard of anything eating a thermometer?"

"No."

Silence.

"Well," I said, "I guess we better do this castration."

"Yeah, I suppose we should."

While we both sympathized with the pig's reluctance to be injected, we had a job to do, and the time for subtle methods was fast dissolving. It was time for the pig snare.

It didn't take any pail of feed to get the pig to come over to us now. He was ready to attack us at any chance he was given. All we had to do was lean in over the fence and the animal would face us with a threatening stance.

We stood by the edge of the pen and shoved the snare in front of his face. On cue he opened his mouth in an effort to eat the snare. Sometimes it's better to keep your mouth closed. With the leading edge of the snare inside his jaws, Darya slid the base of the snare up and tightened the cable around his upper jaw.

The boar froze and let out one ear-shattering bellow. The growing pigs next door, who to this point had shown no interest in our dealings with the boar, rushed to the edge of their pen to get a better look. I climbed back into the pen with the Stresnil and quickly injected the pig.

Darya released the snare and the boar moved off in a huff to the far end of his pen. Now we would just wait for the drug to work.

After twenty minutes we had seen no change in the pig's behaviour.

"Maybe we should read the product insert," Darya suggested.

We sat down on top of an old freezer and started to read the details on this drug that neither of us had much experience with. When we came to the line where it said "not recommended for castrations," both of us stopped.

"I wonder why they say that," Darya said.

"Probably because of what we're seeing. It doesn't work."

Another new plan was needed.

"I say we bite the bullet and castrate him with the snare," I said.

Darya nodded. "There doesn't seem to be much choice. Let's do it."

I filled a bucket with cold water from a nearby tap and added some soap. Darya got the snare back in place and I re-entered the zone.

The snare did its job again and I was able to wash and disinfect the boar's scrotum with little resistance from our patient. With the bucket of water safely back outside the pen, I turned to the surgery.

I pulled back the foil wrapping of the scalpel blade and fashioned it into a handle. I wrapped one hand around the scrotum to tighten a testicle against the skin, then made my incision. Again there was little reaction from the boar, and after pulling the testicle out I applied the emasculator to cut and crush the blood vessels and supporting tissue.

This was working smoothly. One testicle left. Our patient was tolerating this quite well.

I grabbed the second side in the same manner and started the cut. This time the boar let out a grunt and the strength went out of his back legs. He collapsed into the semi-solid manure of his pen with a splash. Just as quickly he jumped back to his feet. But the damage was done: both sides of his scrotum were cut open and both sides were now thoroughly contaminated with manure. All of my careful preparation of the site had been for nothing.

I finished the castration and washed out the wounds the best I could.

Darya and I looked at each other, knowing we were both wondering what else could have gone wrong in this usually routine procedure.

We packed up our gear and went out to see Gord. He was so involved with his sledgehammering that he didn't seem to notice that two vets had taken longer to do this procedure than any unqualified person would normally take.

"How'd it go?"

"Oh . . . not bad. I'll drop in next time I'm by to see how he's doing."

I did drop in about a week later, and I think the boar remembered me. He snorted and charged the edge of his cage. His resilience left no doubt he was one tough pig.

32. Gabby

EVERY FALL, as the air chilled and the leaves changed colour, the artificial ice was installed in the Harbour Grace stadium. From then until spring, I spent one night a week floundering up and down the rink in total bliss.

Hockey has always been a priority in my life, and only important business could keep me away from a game. Sickness usually wasn't a good enough reason. Emergency vet calls occasionally got in the way, but the general rule was that once I was on the ice, I was very hard to find for about an hour.

My teammates would rush about the ice for two minutes and then disintegrate into a mass of quivering hyperventilation on the bench. Hockey is a very anaerobic game. Most players tend to cruise lazily around the ice until they see an opportunity to get hold of the puck. Suddenly they shift from minimal effort to a short burst of all-out exertion. I kept wondering whether some of these guys with decreased fitness levels, but speed and skill remaining from an earlier incarnation, were going to drop over dead from a heart attack.

Chasing cows and two nights a week of karate training kept me in reasonable shape, but I still wasn't above collapsing on the bench after a particularly spirited exertion.

One time, as I was lying back against the wall of our bench after one of these fruitless puck chases, I heard tramping feet approaching from behind. The marching stopped and a familiar roar came from the bleachers behind me.

"Where's Peacock?"

Without turning around, I knew that the speaker was Gabby Wilson. Gabby was of average height and a little more than average girth, with flaming red hair and beard. His rough and hoarse voice probably was related to the fact that he seemed to always be shouting.

The other interesting aspect of Gabby's personality was his utter lack of respect for personal space. Most people are comfortable keeping a few feet away from another person when talking. Gabby didn't seem to understand this nicety of social interaction.

One day, Gabby caught me in the local supermarket while I was helping pick up the week's groceries. He walked up, poked me in the chest with a chubby finger and started to explain how his horse was having breathing problems. We were in the frozen food section, and I kept retreating as Gabby thrust his face into mine. He was wearing a baseball cap, and as he bobbed his head forward for emphasis, he would actually stab me in the forehead with its peak. My retreat eventually backed me up against an open freezer full of turkeys. I leaned back farther and farther into the fowl to escape the onslaught.

Ingrid rounded a corner, deduced my predicament and came to the rescue. It was a relief to play the henpecked husband helping with the groceries if it meant being freed from Gabby's attack.

Back at the hockey rink, Gabby bellowed again, "Where's Peacock?"

I turned and looked up at him and his six assistants. "What do you want?"

"Your woman said that you was down here playing hockey. Come on over to Harv Potter's and have a look at his 'arse. She's got a stoppage of water."

"How long has this been going on?"

"She's been the same for about four hours now."

"If she hasn't changed for that long, she can last another half-hour before we look at her. Sit down and watch the rest of the game."

"Right."

During my next shift on the ice, I looked up into the stands during a lull in play to see Gabby in the uppermost seats surrounded by his gang. Every one of them had a small mountain of french fries smothered in ketchup and a giant tumbler of pop. Gabby was gesticulating wildly and even from down on the ice I could make out enough to tell that he was holding forth on his theories of the origins of different horse maladies.

After the game, I changed quickly and met Gabby and his friends outside the change room door. Everyone seemed to be a little more relaxed. Never underestimate the calming effect of a belly full of french fries and pop.

"Gabby, you and the boys run up to Harv's and make sure the horse is still there and the lights are on. I'll run home and get my truck."

"Right."

I hurried back to Freshwater, gulped a glass of water, pulled on a pair of coveralls and drove the truck over to the barn containing the horse.

Only a small contingent of the experts available to help the horse had made the trek to the stadium. Every equine authority from Harbour Grace was assembled in this one small barn. I wondered if the people left with the horse were concerned about the length of time it had taken Gabby to go down to the stadium and back. Probably not.

I started by asking Harv about what had happened and what had been done so far to help the horse.

Before he could answer, Gabby stepped between us. "Well, Doc, she got into the chicken feed sometime last night and she hasn't eaten a peck since. We've done all the things you should be doin' for an 'arse that's been in chicken feed. You know, Ed put some ginger down into her with a powder horn and stuck an onion up her privates and I rolled a round stick under her belly—"

"It looks like colic, fellas," I interrupted, stepping forward quickly and dramatically pulling my stethoscope from my pocket. "If everybody could just be quiet for a minute, I'll have a listen to her with this."

Gabby seemed not to catch on that he was the only one making any noise. He continued his dissertation on what was wrong with the horse and all the treatments that he had heard of for this kind of problem. Eventually he wandered to a far corner of the barn to sit on a bale of hay, and at last I could hear the horse's heart and lungs.

The horse had a bounding pulse of over fifty beats per

minute and the wild-eyed expression of an animal in great discomfort and fear. Her gums were a healthy pink, but about every minute she would kick at her belly. Through my stethoscope I could hear gurgling sounds in that area. These signs were all consistent with a spasmodic colic brought on by ingestion of too much feed.

Horses with colics generally show signs of abdominal pain and also are often reluctant to pass urine. Many horse owners fix on this last symptom. They call the problem "stoppage of water" and believe it can be cured by forcing the animal to urinate. But colicky horses are reluctant to pass water because their abdomens are too tender for all the abdominal pushing they have to do to empty their bladders. When local horse experts try to cure stoppage of water by putting an onion into a mare's vagina, they do indeed fix the stoppage. The vaginal discomfort overrides the abdominal pain, and the mare passes water. Rather than curing the problem, however, the onion now adds vaginal irritation to the existing colic.

I went out to my truck to pick up a syringe full of painkiller, a gallon of mineral oil, a funnel and a nasogastric tube in a bucket of hot water.

The owner helped me by holding the mare's halter while I slid the needle into the prominent jugular vein running down the neck. After pulling back on the plunger of the syringe and seeing the flash of dull red that reassured me the needle was in the vein, I injected 8 cc's of painkiller. We stepped back from the horse to watch the injection's effect. Within thirty seconds, the wild look in her eyes subsided, the muscles throughout her body visibly relaxed and then she began to eat her hay.

There were oohs and aahs around the barn. Gabby, unswayed in his faith in traditional remedies, was wondering very loudly from his corner whether the stick should have been rolled from left to right rather than from right to left.

The danger when you use painkillers is a false sense of security. The drug turns off the animal's pain sensations but does not deal with the underlying problem. Relieving pain is important and helpful to a colicky horse, but I still had more work to do.

In this case, I was confident that the cause of all of the horse's problems was the ingestion of the chicken feed. A simple solution was to take the feed out of the mare. Bringing the feed back up through the front end isn't practical, and removing it through the side by surgery is a little drastic. The logical way to get rid of the feed is to push it through the back end with a laxative.

It takes a lot of laxative to affect a horse. I usually start with a half a gallon of mineral oil.

Again, I had the owner hold the horse's head as I got my tube out of the hot water. The heat made the plastic tube soft and flexible, and a thin coating of mineral oil made everything slip a whole lot easier. I measured the tube from the horse's nose to the end of her ribs and stuck on a small piece of tape to mark the distance. Horses will not tolerate a tube down their throat the way a cow will and not surprisingly, they often object to plastic tubes being pushed down their noses. I always liked to rub my hand over their eyelids and have a short talk with the horse before we began. Sometimes I wondered if this made me look a little loony, but it seemed to do wonders for relaxing both the vet and the horse.

After our little talk, I rubbed the mare's nose and gently introduced the tube into her left nostril. To the inside of the nostril I could sense an opening that continued on. With a soft push, the tube was in. When the tube was down as far as the tape, I knew that the end was in her stomach. Conveniently, an opening to the hayloft was just in front of the horse's stall. I sent up one of the local experts and had him sit with his legs hanging through the opening. We passed up the funnel and the gallon of mineral oil with instructions to fix the funnel to the end of the tube and pour in half the bottle.

Aside from one false start when then funnel wasn't tightly attached to the tube and a cup of oil found its way down the neck of a spectator, the mineral oil treatment went without incident. The horse looked greatly relieved when the end of the tube was finally removed from her nose. She shook her head and blew out a bit of foul-looking material before putting her head back into the hay.

I explained to the owner to expect some diarrhea soon and to call me if anything worried him about the horse's condition. I could hear Gabby still running on about his great understanding of horses and how they worked.

The next morning Harv called to say that he had found the back of the mare's stall sprayed with slimy manure and that she was looking perfect. The mineral oil had made its way through and likely had taken most of the chicken feed with it. The horse had no more signs of colic, and from then on Harv kept his chicken feed a safer distance from his horse.

A few days later I had stopped in Harbour Grace for gas when a hearty slap on the back and a roar let me know that Gabby had found me again.

"That was great up at Harv's the other night. Yes, boy, it took me some convincin' to tell the boys that they should get the vet and that you could fix up that 'arse. Now if Harv had called me earlier and I had a chance to roll that round stick under her belly before the stoppage of water had really settled in . . ."

"Right."

33. Storm Surgery

NESTLED BETWEEN ROCKY HILLS, the village of Freshwater is one of the most scenic places on an island filled with natural wonders. The hills add a rugged beauty to the views of the ocean and the islands just offshore.

The beauty of Freshwater is, however, stark. It's a place without many trees; the rocks sloping away from the ocean are unshielded from the wind and storms. The village is separated from the nearest larger town, Carbonear, by a road that runs along the rocky shore about a hundred feet above the sea. The severe cliffs falling away from the road make for spectacular scenery, but are completely exposed to any winter storm that may come along.

Most years, at least one blizzard would separate Freshwater from the rest of the world for a few hours or days. When these storms came along, I would have the pleasure of an enforced holiday. There never seemed to be calls when the weather was at its very worst. Perhaps the farmers still had problems but realized that there was no way anyone could get out to help them.

One Easter Sunday, the wind and snow combined to fill the roads into and around Freshwater with deep banks of snow. In places the roads were buried under five or six feet of drifts. Our whole family settled in for a day in the house. In the evening, we enjoyed a leisurely supper and sat together in the living room to read. The wind howled outside and the windows facing the ocean bent in enough that we worried they might implode.

I was well into a wonderful book on how to remain conscious while dreaming, when the phone shook me from my reveries.

"My cow's having trouble calving. You'd better come right away."

I paused to wonder how anyone would think I could get out to see an animal in weather like this. Then I thought I recognized the voice. "Is that you, Mark?"

"Yep. I think you better get over here right now."

Mark Marshall was a quiet man. He seldom called and was the only client in my practice that I could possibly see that day. He lived just over a quarter of a mile from my house in the same village. If it turned out I couldn't drive to Mark's barn, I could still walk.

"I'll be there in a minute, Mark."

It seemed my reading was done for the night. While the rest of the family read in the warmth of the living room, I put on my coveralls and boots.

Mats was almost always frantic to get outside to go on vet calls, so when he ran up the stairs as I reached for the door, I knew this weather wasn't going to be pleasant. The instant I stepped out the front door, my suspicions were verified. Driving snow took my breath away when I faced into the wind. The snow was piled nearly two feet deep in front of the truck. I climbed up into the cab and sat wondering whether I should attempt the drive across the village or set off on foot.

The storm limited visibility, but from what I could see, the road between my house and Mark's barn was fairly free of snow. The truck started with the first turn of the key and with a loud clunk it lurched forward. Somewhere down under the vehicle something had broken free of ice.

I really couldn't see much, and getting through the piles of snow on the road required considerable momentum. This combination of poor visibility and high speed made for an exciting trip. The wind and snow would let up for an instant, and if I saw deep snow ahead I would press harder on the gas. Every time it hit a new drift, the truck would buck and then threaten to come to a halt. Eventually, though, I managed to cover the short distance to Mark's barn. With no one on the road and no places to pull in, I left the truck in the middle of the little-used lane in front of the barn.

Holding my breath, I stepped out into the blizzard again and collected my calving gear from the back of the truck. The wind wrestled with me for control of the barn door, and once I managed to pry the door open a crack, a sharp gust grabbed it from my hand and smashed it against the outside wall. After placing my equipment well into the barn, I returned my attention to the door, where Mark joined me. The violent beating that the door had taken must have shifted the hinges, because once I heaved it back into the door frame, it didn't fit properly. Seeing how the door now banged into the frame, Mark found a piece of baler twine and tied the door handle to a post inside the barn. The door lurched like a panicking trapped animal, but we were now separated from the storm.

"Nice night, Mark."

"It's lovely, boy."

Despite our attempts at levity, he was right. It was lovely. The barn had that rich smell of hay and animal that makes small, clean barns so inviting. The three cows in the barn kept the building at a pleasant temperature. Two of them were pulling hanks of hay from the piles in front of them and chewing contentedly. They didn't seem the least perturbed by the arrival of another human—or by their stallmate panting on the ground. Steam rose from her sides, and every few seconds she would tense her whole body and push.

Mark had a bucket of warm water ready for me, so I started by reaching up inside the cow to assess the situation. Immediately, I felt the calf's head. I could tell just with my hand that this was one big calf. "This calf's a monster, Mark. We're going to have to do some cutting here."

"Suppose this is going to be expensive."

"It'll probably be cheaper than if you had to have a plumber come out tonight, and I'm sure it'll be cheaper than losing a cow and a calf. Ready to start?"

"Suppose we should."

I shaved the side of the cow and scrubbed up the site with iodine soap. It was surprising how rarely a cow would get infected as a result of surgery carried out in such basic conditions. When operating in a barn, I would make every effort to maintain cleanliness, but to suggest that conditions even approached sterility would be laughable. No matter how carefully I shaved and scrubbed, hair always found its way into the area being operated on. The barns were filled with dust, and it wasn't uncommon for a big piece of dirt to work its way loose from the ceiling and fall right into a surgical site.

I froze the side of the cow with injections of lidocaine and sat on a bale to wait for the drug to take effect.

"Ever seen one of these done before, Mark?"

"Nope, and I don't like blood much."

"Don't worry about that. There won't be much blood. We'll be done in no time."

Once the freezing had been given a chance to work, it was time to start the surgery. Blasts of wind shook the barn and the door rattled as I scrubbed up and pulled out a scalpel. The first cut through the skin was looking good. With the right amount of pressure, I was through the skin and well into the muscles when I heard Mark.

"Oh man . . ."

I glanced over my shoulder to see him stumble toward the door with both hands clutching the sides of his head. He undid the twine holding the door closed and just as it exploded outward he crumpled to the floor.

A lot of things had to be dealt with at once. Both the cow and the barn door were open. The open door was quickly making the barn less comfortable to work in, and the open cow required my full attention. On top of this, I had a farmer who I hoped had only fainted.

Mark was my first priority. The surgery could wait for a short while, so I put my scalpel down on a clean sheet and hurried over to my stricken assistant.

I placed my hand on his shoulder. "You okay, Mark?"

He moaned and sat up. "Oh man, this is embarrassing. I've got to get to the house."

I had visions of Mark falling again out in the blizzard with no one to see him go down. This could turn into a serious mess. Reaching out into the storm, I caught hold of the door and yanked it closed. A few quick half hitches of baler twine kept the blizzard outside.

"I don't think that's a good idea, Mark. You'd better stay here with me. Sit down on this bale and look the other away. We can talk while I get this done and you can head back inside when we're finished."

Mark stood and rubbed his hands across the sides of his head. This took some of the hay out of his hair, but he still had a good covering of vegetation.

"Okay, I'll sit here."

"That's great. We can have a chat."

I washed my hands again and picked up the scalpel. My first cut had opened a vertical incision into the skin nearly eighteen inches long. I estimated that this opening would be large enough to get out the calf that I had felt inside.

As I sliced through the remaining muscles under the skin, I noticed a slight twitching of the fibres, but the cow remained unconcerned.

"Did you see the Leafs last night?"

Mark was a diehard Toronto Maple Leafs fan, and I figured that the topic might keep him occupied. I was only a casual fan myself.

"Whaddaya mean? Toronto didn't play last night."

So much for my attempts to present myself as someone capable of talking about hockey. But fortunately my ignorance wasn't going to keep a true believer from discussing his passion.

"They beat Detroit the night before. That was some game. You should have seen . . ."

This monologue was what I was hoping for. I didn't mind talking a little as I worked, but my preference was to put at least the majority of my concentration on the work I was doing.

With the muscles all cut, it was time to enter the body cavity. The abdomen of a mammal is closed in by a thin sheet of tissue known as the peritoneum. This sheet keeps the insides of an animal sterile and away from the dirt of the outside world. Once inside the peritoneum, cleanliness takes on a new significance.

With one slice, I opened the peritoneum from one end of the skin incision to the other. The opening of this protected part of the cow was attended with a slight sucking sound and then a soft waft of warm air. The air from the inside of a living animal has a subtle smell that feels like life and death at the same time. The odour is vital and filled with life, but at the same time it brings a suggestion of meat.

With the peritoneum open, I could see an expanse of smooth white tissue in front of me. This was the rumen, the largest stomach. The uterus that contained the calf would be just behind it.

I washed my hands and arms again in the iodine solution in my pail. Mark's commentary had come to a halt.

"How ya doin', Mark?"

"Not bad. I was just thinkin' about whether I should buy a trailer."

"Tell me about trailers. Why would you want one?"

"Well, the wife and I travels quite a bit and I figure it would be cheaper to have one of those RV rigs than stayin' in hotels . . ."

He was off on another discourse and I had more time to work uninterrupted. An occasional "Hmm" or "You're kidding" was enough to keep him going.

I reached in behind the rumen and felt the uterus. I ran my hand along the two horns of this organ, and was sure that there was only one calf. With the calf as big as it was, there was really no need for a sibling.

I cupped my hand under the portion of the uterus with the calf inside and rocked it up and forward until it appeared in the incision. The visible portion contained the back legs of the calf.

My plan was to cut this part of the uterus and then pull the calf out by the back legs. Normally at this point I would get some assistance from a farmer, but I wanted to keep Mark out of this as long as I could. With a little more manipulation, I was able to tip the ends of the calf's legs inside the uterus out over the edge of my opening.

I stabilized the uterus in position with one hand and cut in toward the calf with the other. Then I put the scalpel down and reached inside. I now had a good hold on the calf's hind legs. But my arms weren't long enough to pull the calf all the way out *and* keep the opened uterus from slipping back into the abdomen.

"Mark, how you doin'?"

"Not so bad."

"I'm going to need some help from you now."

"Oh man."

"All the cutting is done, don't worry. All I'd like you to do is pull the calf out. Can you do that?"

"I guess so."

"Well, come over here."

"Oh man."

Mark rose from his bale and turned toward me and the cow. I worried for a second that he might collapse again and that I would be in a worse situation than if I hadn't called him. To my relief, he came over without hesitation and took the calf's legs from me.

"Okay, now pull slowly and steadily."

As Mark pulled, I held on to the uterus and watched his eyes. The full back legs and then the hips emerged from the side of the cow. With another tug, the chest and shoulders were in view, and then without warning the full calf fell from the incision to the ground with a splat.

"It's a heifer and she's a beauty." Mark's squeamishness disappeared as he examined his new calf.

"Get her dried off a bit," I told him, "and pull her up to the mother so she can lick her off."

Mark eagerly complied and I started to close the cow. Two layers of absorbable suture put the uterus back together and another line shut the peritoneum. More stitches in the muscles pulled the hole in the cow's side back together, and a single row of nylon stitches closed the skin. Other than a foot-and-a-half-long line of stitches running down her shaved side, the cow looked as good as new.

With an iodine dip for the calf's navel and a shot of hormone to help shrink down the cow's uterus, the job was finished.

If it was possible, it sounded like the storm outside had gained momentum. I told Mark that we would worry about the bill for this later. It would be a simple matter to come down to his house when the weather was reasonable and straighten out our accounts.

Once all my equipment was cleaned and dried, I stashed it into my case. Mark was looking fine, and I wasn't worried about leaving him alone. All worries about the night's work had dissolved with the appearance of his new calf. He didn't look like he would be heading back to the house soon.

Now I had to get home. When I stepped outside, I could see that new mounds of snow had appeared since I'd arrived. The truck was now ensheathed in snow up to the windows. There was no chance that I was driving home that night. I stowed my gear in the back, locked the doors and set off for home.

A stroll of about a quarter mile through a village as beautiful as Freshwater is usually an enjoyable diversion. But in this storm there was nothing pleasant about the walk home. The wind and snow were blasting directly into my face. I couldn't walk upright. Only by putting my head down or by facing away from the wind could I catch my breath. I made my way along the lane in front of Mark's barn. The road was filled in with three feet of snow. It was exhausting work, and when I reached the main road, I stopped with my back to the wind and caught my breath.

The best way home was to sprint between the houses along the way. I ran as quickly as I could to the first house and leaned against its leeward side. Just ahead I could see the light shining out through the windows of Clayton's house. The place looked warm and inviting. Our family had spent many pleasant evenings there, but I knew that stopping in anywhere would only prolong the difficulty of this trip.

With the shelter of four houses, I reached the final hundred-yards stretch to home. All that was left was to cross the bridge above the beach and climb a final short ascent to our house. The road turned sharply so the wind would no longer be in my face.

This seemed at first to simplify movement, but I soon found that the gusts were strong enough to blow me sideways as I walked. As I passed Max's place, I reflected on how neighbours like him had helped with the renovations that had made our house stormproof. By bending over, I was able to stay on track and covered the final distance to my front door.

Despite the howling wind and crashing waves, it was easy to sleep that night. I was exhausted from the work and the difficult trip home. Thinking that there was enough snow to keep the village snowed in at least through the morning, I was in no hurry to get up the next day.

At about nine o'clock I was surprised to hear a snowplow rumbling along the road. I hurried to put on my warmest clothes and headed outside. The storm was over, and we had a beautiful cold, sunny day ahead. The sun set diamonds sparkling off the snow as I easily covered the short distance that had given me so much difficulty the night before.

As I neared Mark's barn, I saw that the snowplow had already cleared the lane. The plow had taken two passes and left my truck in the middle of the road. The truck was standing on over two feet of snow.

I climbed up into the truck and drove down off the pile of snow, leaving behind a white cubic monument to the adventure of the night before.

34. What Happened to the Seal

MOST OF MY WORK WITH wildlife involved animals that lived on the land. Occasionally visitors from the sea would also need a hand.

Often when investigating a sick animal, I would look at a sample of its blood under a microscope. Preparing blood slides was difficult and monotonous. A fresh drop of blood had to be scraped across a slide with the end of another slide. To ensure a smear of the right thickness, the drop had to be just the right size and the slides had to be pulled across each other at the right speed and angle.

I was throwing out my third poor attempt on a sample from an anemic horse when Sharon called down the hall that I was wanted on the phone. It was a relief to get away from the blood.

A woman from Harbour Grace was on the phone telling me a sick seal was on the beach near the *Kyle*. My first reaction was to suggest that there was nothing necessarily wrong with a seal just because it was sitting on a beach. When she added that the seal had been there for four days, I became more interested. I told her I would have a look.

In Canada, wildlife living on land is the responsibility of the provincial governments. I was a provincial government employee and so had no problem working on land-based wildlife. Marine mammals such as seals, however, are a federal responsibility. Federal law requires permits and permission before anyone can have much to do with them.

With this in mind, I thought it might be wise to give Fisheries a call.

"Hello, bonjour, Fisheries, how can I help you?"

"I'd like to talk to somebody about a seal."

"Inspector Pinnipé is off on training this month, but you can pick up a sealing licence at our office."

"Well, I'm not really interested in shooting one. I'm a vet and I just wanted to make sure it was okay for me to look at one in Harbour Grace and maybe treat it if I need to."

"Let me just look in our directory here, sir." There was a long pause. "You still there, sir? Okay, if you take down this number you can phone the Marine Mammal Response Program in Ottawa and I'm sure they can deal with this problem."

My attempt to help this seal wasn't really a problem until I had phoned the Fisheries office. I dutifully took down the number and thought to myself that I had gone deep enough into this mire of bureaucracy. If this seal was going to get any help from me, it would have to be without government sanction. If someone wanted to complain, I would deal with it later.

I drove down to Harbour Grace and parked on the side of the road within sight of the *Kyle*. The *Kyle* is an old steamer that is grounded in the shallows at the head of Harbour Grace harbour. The *Kyle* had an illustrious history as a supply boat and sealing vessel from the time of the First World War until the 1960s. When she reached the end of her useful life, she was brought to Harbour Grace to be sunk in the near off-shore depths. A storm that blew up before she could be scuttled left her the stranded tourist attraction—or eyesore—that she is today.

It took me a while to find the seal. She was down over a small bank about fifty yards from the edge of the highway. This was a harbour seal, about five feet long and weighing about two hundred pounds. She made no reaction as I scrabbled noisily along the rocks toward her. She seemed to be sleeping. She had a sleek and shining black coat with slate-coloured splotches all over.

I touched her back flippers with my boot. Still no reaction. I reached down and touched the seal's back. The full animal jerked into action. Pushing down with her flippers and arching her back, the seal reared up and spun around to face me. I backed away from the hissing mouth with its surprisingly long canine teeth.

This was an unusual kind of physical examination, but now I knew this animal was aware of its surroundings and could move. I could see no obvious injuries, and other than the fact that she had been sitting on land longer than usual, nothing seemed untoward. Perhaps it would help to chase the animal back into the water.

With the seal facing me, I made a feint toward it with my arms in the air. The seal moved toward me and let out an intimidating roar. Evidently I wouldn't be chasing her anywhere. I then wondered if it was possible to get her to chase me. I moved around behind the seal, reached out again and touched her on the back. This time there was no reaction. It was almost as though she knew I was trying to get her to turn around. I rubbed her back a little farther up, but not too close to her mouth and those teeth. The seal's reaction was to put her head down and relax.

There was no more I could do, so I went off on other calls. On the way home in the evening, I stopped again to have a look at the seal. She was in the same place and appeared to be resting comfortably.

The next morning I stopped by again. There was no change, except she had moved a little farther in from the shore. She was now up over the small ridge I had found her behind. It was now easy to see her from the road.

Two days later I got a phone call from a marine mammal researcher from the university in St. John's. He wondered if I had heard of or seen the seal. I explained that I had been checking a couple of times a day for a while and I hadn't seen anything obviously wrong. He said he would like to come out with a few people the next day.

I arrived at the seal scene half an hour before our appointed time, thinking that I might get another look at the animal before too many people were around. When I pulled up under the gaze of the *Kyle*, I saw the university truck parked well off the road next to the seal.

The researcher was holding one end of a tape measure. As he jumped around the seal calling out numbers, a young student held the other end at the tip of the seal's hind flippers. Two more students with clipboards were furiously writing down every measurement the researcher called out. I was disappointed to see that the seal wasn't making much effort to chase away this intrusion on her dignity. Perhaps she was getting worse.

The researcher wore a bright orange survival suit; it was bulky and cumbersome but was guaranteed to keep the wearer warm on a chilly morning such as this one. The students were all young women, their bright, clean rain jackets and pants didn't look like they had seen much action. Their up-to-the-minute-cool Peruvian toques suggested style and appearance was a priority. I felt a little out of place in my drab coveralls and dull barn coat. Stylistically I had more in common with the local I spotted sitting on a rock next to the seal watching the proceedings. His soiled oilskin suit and the way his cap was tipped back on his head marked him as someone who knew something of the sea. The cigarette hanging from his lower lip finished off the picture. He leaned back on his elbows with an amused expression.

The researcher turned when I approached.

"Hey, Doc, how's it goin'? Great day, isn't it?"

"It's lovely. You getting some measurements?" I was always ready with a keen question that added to my knowledge of the situation.

"Yep. Anything you want here?"

"I'd love to get this girl's temperature and a little blood to have a look at. A sample would give us a better idea if there's anything wrong with her and if we can give her anything that might help."

"No sweat. Hey, Stan, can you grab hold of the seal for the vet?"

The man I had assumed was a local bystander flicked his cigarette away and stood. He brought his hands together behind his back and slowly raised them in a subtle stretch. In the back of the university van he found a section of cargo netting about two yards square. With the net over his shoulder he made a slow walk around the seal. It surprised the rest of us watching as much as the seal when he threw the net from behind and with an efficient leap landed on her back. This obviously wasn't the first time he'd wrangled a seal.

The seal roared in surprise, but soon settled when she saw there was no escaping from this man. I got in close as soon as the seal stopped her thrashing and inserted a rectal thermometer. This was the easy part.

Seals are fat. Most of their body is encased in a layer of fat that allows them to live in the cold waters of the North Atlantic. But this blubber also makes it difficult to get at blood vessels. The reading I had done suggested that the best place to take a blood sample was from the veins that run through the vertebrae or the veins of the hind flippers.

The idea of sticking a needle in close to the spinal cord of a wild animal that might flail at any moment didn't appeal to me. Paralysis from an unnecessary procedure was a risk that I wasn't willing to take.

The second option didn't sound easy, though. The veins that run among the equivalent of toes in a seal's hind flippers are quite small and they can't be seen through the skin. When I touched the needle to the seal's flipper, she squirmed just enough to make it impossible to find a small vein. I asked the researcher to hold the flipper solidly against the ground.

The next time I touched the needle to the skin, the seal roared and thrashed.

At that point, I decided that a blood sample likely wouldn't give us enough useful information to be worth the seal's discomfort. I would have to be satisfied with some observations of heart and breathing rate, temperature and a fecal sample. I discussed the situation with the researcher, and we agreed that there wasn't much obviously wrong with the seal.

The next morning I swung by to take a look at the seal before going into the office. I could see no sign of her from the road, so I parked the truck and scoured the area. She was gone. It was a relief to think that she had made up her mind to head back home. Perhaps our work the previous day had convinced her that life in the ocean was preferable to the "help" she was getting from us.

Back at the office I was telling the guys at work how I had been involved in scaring the seal back into the sea, when Sharon called me to the phone. It was the CBC calling from St. John's, wanting to know if I would do an interview with them about the seal in Harbour Grace. Sensing that this was a feel-good success story, I happily agreed.

The radio host started by asking me why I thought Newfoundlanders couldn't leave seals alone. I patiently explained that I didn't share that opinion. He went on to ask what I made of all the people who had harassed the seal. Again I bit my tongue and carefully said that I hadn't seen any evidence of anyone bothering the seal. I told him I had been visiting this seal at least twice a day since it came ashore and in all that time had never seen anyone bothering the seal.

I didn't mention that the worst harassment I had seen was myself trying to collect blood.

I was surprised when the interview ended with no questions having been asked about what might have been wrong with the animal and what my impressions as a veterinarian were. The host told me to listen the next morning around eight o'clock to hear the interview.

Listening to yourself being interviewed on the radio involves a level of masochism. You know you'll be disappointed. I always wonder if I really sound as bad as that, and I always think of clever things I could have said in response to every question.

In the lead-up to the seal interview, the radio host said that he would be playing a tape of conversations with the mayor of the town and a representative from the local police. I thought it was odd that they didn't say anything about the local vet.

There was no interview with the vet. The mayor said it was too bad that people had harassed the poor seal. The police spokesman regretted that the animal had suffered grave injury from the locals, while emphasizing that only a few people had been involved. I supposed that my talk didn't fit the sensational story the radio station was trying to peddle. I was only mildly disappointed—until the police spokesman said: "This unfortunate seal was in such poor condition that one of our officers had to dispatch it with his sidearm."

I couldn't believe what I was hearing. I had seen this animal within a few hours of when it was "dispatched" and there was nothing wrong with her as far as I could see. Some expert from the police force had decided that the seal was better off dead.

With rising anger I headed off to the police station. The lobby seemed designed to intimidate. A room lined with concrete blocks was filled with posters of wanted felons and lost children. A bulletproof window had a small opening at the bottom to pass fines and papers through. A solid-looking metal door led to the offices beyond.

Every time I had come to this building before, the mood set by the lobby had made me feel small and in awe of the power of the police. Not this time.

A secretary came to the glass. "Can I help you, sir?"

"I want to talk to whoever shot the seal."

"Why would you want that, sir?"

"I'm a vet and that was my patient. Someone shot my patient."

"Just a second, sir." The woman went away to the back offices.

After a few minutes an older officer came to the window. He had wire-framed glasses pushed well down over his nose and a belly that threatened to cover the firearm conspicuously belted to his side.

He peered at me through the glass. "Are you the vet, sir?"

"I am. Why did you guys shoot the seal?"

"That seal was very sick, sir. We put it out of its misery."

It was taking every effort to remain civil. "What was it that made you believe it was sick? Did you examine that seal? I've been seeing that seal twice a day for the last week and examining her every day. I didn't see anything that made me think she was sick. I like to think I know a bit about sick animals, that's my job. How did you know it was sick?"

"Well, sir, actually the animal was a hazard to traffic."

"What?"

"Traffic was being held up because people were slowing down to look at the seal."

I had heard enough. I turned to leave, but stopped with one more thought. I turned back. "What happened to the seal?"

"It was buried, sir."

"Tell me where she was buried. I'm digging her up and I'm doing a post-mortem."

He hesitated. "The seal is buried just outside the dump. There's a pile of rocks just to the left of the main gate."

I left the station more disappointed and angry than when I arrived. Nothing could be done for the seal now. No one would say anything about the seal being shot. After all, this was a federal animal, and it was a federal police officer who had shot her.

After driving home to pick up a shovel, I made my way to the dump and found the burial site. There was the pile of rocks, just in front of a sign warning citizens of serious fines for leaving material outside the dump fence. I wondered who would give out these fines.

It didn't take much work to unearth the seal. She was in the proverbial shallow grave; it seemed appropriate for her shady demise. I opened the grave a little wider than it had been dug so I could open the carcass.

I carefully went over every inch of skin looking for evidence of trauma. When I found nothing on the outside I skinned the animal. If people had been throwing rocks at the seal I was sure there would be some evidence of bruising on the inside of the skin. The only unusual finding I saw was two neat holes through the skin over the head. These were from bullets.

I drew a small portion of blood from within the heart. Now I had the sample I had been looking for before. The organs all looked normal, but I took small tissue samples from the vital organs and put them in bottles filled with formaldehyde. These would be sent to the University of Prince Edward Island to be examined microscopically by veterinary pathologists.

When I started looking along the digestive tract, I was surprised to feel that the stomach was heavy and filled with very hard objects. I cut through the stomach wall and was surprised to discover seven large stones inside the stomach. Some of the stones were as large as softballs. It was hard to imagine how the seal had swallowed these. I didn't see anything else unusual inside the seal.

Later, I phoned around to people across North America who knew much more than me about seals. One vet from Florida who worked in a marine park told me that she sometimes saw seals that had eaten large rocks. She wasn't sure whether this was an indication of disease or boredom or just some natural attempt to straighten out their ability to ballast.

I'll never know why the seal climbed up on the beach, but I know it wasn't rocks from the outside or inside that killed her.

35. The SPCA at Christmas

PERHAPS THE MOST CHALLENGING part of vet work is investigating animal abuse. Sometimes these were horrifically abused or unbelievably neglected animals. Sometimes it was just a case of a disgruntled neighbour and an outraged owner. Nevertheless, every case seemed to bring out the worst in people.

Two weeks before Christmas one year the St. John's branch of the SPCA called me to report that a dog in Bay Roberts was not being properly fed and was often left alone. Would I go and have a look at it? Because I never knew how serious these cases were, I often left them until I was in the same area for farm calls. But when nearly a week passed without a farm animal needing help in the vicinity of Bay Roberts, I thought I should make a special trip.

It was a beautiful sunny day as Mats and I left the office and climbed into the truck—and one of those rare windless days in Newfoundland. The woodsmoke rising vertically from chimneys was a visual delight. I listened to a fascinating program on the radio about a man who collected musical instruments from around the globe. All was well with the world. The trip to Bay Roberts passed quickly. My directions said that the dog was at the third-last house on the main road.

This part of town was well-to-do. Yet the house I pulled up at broke the monotony of the upper-middle-class ones all around. It was small, a one-storey bungalow that could have used a paint job and some new shingles five years ago. When I turned in the drive, I was enjoying the radio so much that I was more than a little reluctant to turn it off and leave the truck. I rubbed Mats's head as I stepped down from the cab. He immediately shifted from the passenger seat to the throne next to it.

A doghouse stood in front of where I had parked the truck. As I stepped forward, a medium-sized dog tentatively poked its nose out the door. I knelt down and whistled softly.

"Come here, fella."

The dog leapt from its house and sprinted toward me. It is amazing how much can run through your head in a second or two. I wondered if calling the dog had been a good idea. Was he friendly? Was he going to bite me? Why had I knelt down in a position that I couldn't get out of quickly?

My musings were interrupted when the dog violently reached the end of his rope. He brought up with a lurch and fell to the ground coughing. As he recovered from this rude intrusion on his intended visit, he sat up and panted. His eyes sparkled in an unmistakably friendly manner and he stroked the air with one front paw.

I stepped forward and rubbed his side. The dog flipped over on his back and revelled in the attention I gave him. Out of the corner of my eye I could see Mats standing with both front feet on the steering wheel, his head cocked in disbelief.

With the dog sprawled on his back, I noted that he was a little thin and his coat could use a bit more combing, but otherwise he was in reasonable shape. Dogs are forgiving creatures, so his friendly demeanour was no proof that he was being given attention.

It surprised me that no one had come out of the house to see what I was doing playing with their dog. Smoke was rising from the chimney, so someone had to be home.

I headed over to the back door of the house and knocked. The muffled din of a daytime soap leaked through the walls, so I banged a second and third time.

I began to think that perhaps whoever lived in the house had just popped out for a minute, and I decided to wait in the truck. But just as I backed away from the step, I heard footsteps approaching. The door slowly opened.

A middle-aged woman, clasping the door close to her body with both hands, showed just half of her face. She looked fragile and haggard. Her hair was thin, grey and untended.

"Mornin', ma'am. How are you today?"

"Okay . . ." She clutched the door closer.

"I'm just here looking at your dog."

"Don't take him. He's all I got."

"Don't worry, I'm not going to take your dog. Do you like your dog?"

"I loves him. He's all I got."

"Do you ever take him for a walk?"

"Sometimes."

"Do you think you could take him out every day?"

"I will. Please don't take my doggie."

"Listen, no one is taking your dog. I'm not here to hurt you or your dog. I just want to help you make sure he's happy."

She opened the door to look out at her pet. The eye that had been hidden was surrounded by a swollen purple mass with a green tinge. She was wearing a dirty old nightgown, and I was sure I saw scars on her forearms.

There was certainly abuse at this address, but the dog was likely the lucky one. I asked her a few more questions about her pet and suggested she feed him some proper dog food along with his usual table scraps. She promised to take him for more walks and comb him from time to time.

As I walked back to the truck, I saw her next-door neighbour leaning against the side of his nearly new top-of-the-line recreational vehicle.

"Hey, you here checkin' out that dog?"

"Yeah."

"'Bout time—I called in about that weeks ago. Those people got no business havin' a dog. They got no business livin' here."

I didn't answer and climbed back into my truck.

There was a commotion on the road as I manoeuvred the truck around. The local Christmas parade was just coming down the hill, and I would have to wait for it to pass.

The decorated cars and trucks, the cheerleaders, the bands and Santa Claus in the back of a pickup all passed by. Only one vehicle drew any reaction from me. An undecorated flatbed truck was covered with men holding bags. Most of them held a bottle of beer. As they passed by me, one passenger slurred out, "Have some candy, buddy," and tossed a handful of candy against my windshield.

I sat quietly in the truck for over a minute after the parade had passed, and then I turned to Mats and ruffled his fur.

"Come on, buddy, let's go pick up a bag of dog food."

36. This Is Your Home

I LOOKED FORWARD TO THE weekends when I had no calls so I could work on our house. We had redone the inside, built an extension with big windows looking out on the ocean and nailed new clapboard all around.

It was a beautiful crisp and sunny morning with a golden carpet of leaves in the front yard and a few more still up in the trees. The lower parts of the house were already painted, and I was at the top of a ladder finishing the last touches near the eaves.

Painting can be delightfully mindless work; it's possible to drift off to other places and still do a serviceable job of putting on colour. Down below I could see Adrian and Astrid throwing a basketball at the hoop on our garage. Liam was talking with our next-door neighbour and surrogate grandmother, Olga. We had come a long way from our early days in the village, when Olga had suggested that she'd have us in for a meal if we weren't so "stuck up being doctors and all." I was in the middle of blissful reveries when a loud commotion from down the hill interrupted my trance. Two men were shouting to a neighbour three houses along, and I could distinctly hear her say, "Go get Andrew."

In my work it wasn't unusual to see people in complete panic. Often it's a dog or a cat that someone has hit with a car, and many times it means a lot of work. I had a morning's painting planned and a full schedule for the afternoon, and I wasn't looking forward to spending a good part of this beautiful fall day in surgery.

The two men charged up to my front yard. They stopped to catch their breath and leaned on the gate post for support. "There's a boat tipped over in the cove and three guys in the water. Can you get your kayak?"

I don't think it really happened this way, but I have this vision of myself leaping into action from the top of the extension ladder by placing my hands and boots on the outsides of the ladder and sliding down to the ground at a furious rate.

There is no time to waste when people fall into the ocean. This is especially true in Newfoundland, where the waters are chilled by the frigid Labrador current flowing down from the north. All of us understood that we must get to the men in the water as soon as possible.

We ran around to the back of the house to the kayak storage area. The door was fastened with a combination lock, and in the mad rush the lock was difficult to operate. It went through my mind to take a hammer to the whole latch as I fumbled with the tumblers. After a few frustrating seconds that seemed more like minutes, the lock sprang free.

As the two men hurried away with the kayak, I grabbed a paddle and yelled at the girls to bring out some life jackets. They had already sensed the urgency of the situation, and they rushed inside, gathered up the jackets and brought them to the side door.

It's amazing how fast you can run with work boots and painting coveralls on while carrying a paddle and three life preservers. It's even more amazing how fast two men can move with a seventeen-foot ocean-going kayak under their arms. As I started down the road for the cove, the men with the kayak were in front of me, and I don't think I gained a foot on them during the run.

At the beach I assembled the paddle, put two life preservers under the bungee cords behind the cockpit and launched into the sea. There was some chop on the surface and a little swell, but the water could hardly be described as rough.

It didn't take long to paddle out the couple hundred yards to where the small boat was capsized. As I approached I saw Clayton, Clarence and Frank, three good friends and some of the most experienced fishermen of the community, clutching their inverted and submerged boat, holding it tightly to a buoy. Somewhere from the back of my head a rule from all of the swimming and lifesaving courses I had taken rose to consciousness. Never make contact with victims in the water unless necessary and minimize the possibility of their drowning you. Good idea. I pulled the kayak up about ten feet from the accident site.

"How's it going, guys?"

"We're some glad to see you out here," Clarence said. "It's getting a bit cold and Frank can't swim."

My first assessment of the situation was that other than embarrassment they weren't suffering too much from their ordeal. Everyone seemed quite relaxed and I could see no signs of hypothermia. The nonswimmer was the least of my worries, as he had a life jacket on.

"How am I going to get you guys in? I can throw you life jackets and tow you back one at a time or everybody can come back together."

"There's a rope on the stern of this boat," Clayton said. "Take it and tow the whole works back into shore."

This struck me as a reasonable plan, so I had them throw me the length of rope and I tied it around my waist. With the line attached directly to my body, I felt that I would be aware of how well my cargo was following. With the knife attached to my life jacket, I would be able to quickly remove the rope if anything went wrong.

The load was a little difficult to get moving, but we were soon making reasonable progress toward shore. With every stroke of the paddle the rope cut into me a little, but as long as I kept paddling hard, we all moved along quite steadily.

As we headed toward the shore, a large crowd congregated to watch the proceedings. Cars lined the road, children ran up and down the rocky coastline, and half the adult population of the village joined in the festive occasion.

I noticed three men running toward the water with a small green boat in their arms. It was a strange craft, about three feet by five feet, with square corners, flat ends and shallow sides. It looked more like a coffin than a boat, and it seemed like a boat or coffin that I wouldn't want anything to do with. As they reached the slipway, two of the men started climbing into this odd vessel. I was unsure how they intended to propel their boat, as neither man had a paddle. One of them did have a piece of plank in his hands.

My passengers started to yell at the men in the green boat. They ordered them to get away from it and suggested that they were somewhat less than sane to put two people into such a small vessel. The spectators picked up the refrain, and the men with the boat soon agreed that it wouldn't be safe for two of them to go out.

The man without a plank jumped out and pushed the remaining man and the boat out into the ocean. It made an interesting diversion from my paddling to watch this fellow with his nearly useless paddle and only slightly better boat attempt to navigate the waves. I couldn't guess what he intended to do when and if he reached us. I wondered if I'd have to pluck an extra victim from the sea.

By the time the small boat drew near to us, the three men in the water had assessed the seaworthiness of this new arrival and decided that it posed great risk to the success of our operation. They threatened the new rescuer with all types of bodily harm if he attempted to touch either their boat or the kayak. Newfoundland English is always imaginative, and I was treated to a fascinating array of adjectives to describe both the boat and its pilot. With some relief we watched the green boat turn around and begin a zigzag course back to the shore.

As I neared the shore, one of the spectators waded out to the kayak and took the rope from around my waist. I paddled out of the way as a group of men pulled the upside-down boat and three bedraggled fishermen onto dry land.

As the fuss died down and the crowd began to disperse, I came ashore and climbed out of the kayak. Clarence walked over to where I was standing.

"There was some ice in the bottom of the boat," he explained, "and I slipped over to the low side when Clayt started hauling up the anchor. Thanks for pulling us out of the water. It's lucky you were around."

It was a thrill to think that I had helped out my neighbours. From time to time I was able to be of minor assistance with their cats and dogs, but I felt I could never match the support they gave to me.

Since we had moved to Freshwater, our neighbours had been nothing but supportive. They helped us fix up our house, they babysat our children and they had us in for meals. We couldn't imagine living among better people.

Liam had come down to the beach to watch the morning's activity and he helped me carry the kayak back up to the house. On the way he mentioned that Olga had asked the family to come over for fish and brewis for lunch.

We poked the kayak back into its shed and cleaned up. Ingrid, Liam, Adrian, Astrid and I all headed down to Olga's. She met us at the door.

"It's a good thing you have that kayak what with the rest of the boats being pulled out of the water for the year. The boys were in trouble out there."

It was great to hear a positive comment about my kayak. Usually I got anything from gentle ribbing to outright derision when I headed out on the ocean in my diminutive craft.

"Come on in and sit down, the fish is ready."

We all pulled in to the table eager to get into a great meal of potatoes, onions, salt cod, hard bread and the surprisingly delicious fried pork fat cubes called scrunchions. It didn't seem that long ago that I wouldn't have known what salt fish was.

"This is delicious, Olga," I said. "We never had this kind of food at home."

She put down her fork and looked at me for a second. "What are you talking about, home? Sure your kids were all born here, you're one of us. This *is* your home."

ACKNOWLEDGEMENTS

For *Creatures of the Rock* to happen, the stories had to be lived and then they had to be written. I have been very fortunate to have had a great deal of help throughout both of these adventures. While it would be impossible to mention all the mentors and friends who should be thanked, I will list a few.

None of this would have been possible without the wonderful clients and animals I've seen since I started practising veterinary medicine in Newfoundland. If I have ever attended to your dog, cat, horse, cow or moose, you and your charges are a part of this story. Thank you for your support throughout the years.

The people of Freshwater made Ingrid and I feel welcome from the moment we first saw this delightful village. Thanks for the friendship and tea.

The veterinarians who practised farm animal medicine during my time in Newfoundland were always helpful. Special thanks must go out to Hugh Whitney, Ron Taylor, Ron Dunphy, Doug Tweedie, Robert Hudson and the late Alton Smith. I have been privileged to have such outstanding colleagues. My friends at Salmonier Nature Park were always a pleasure to work with. A heartfelt thank you to Sharon Bavis for three decades of patience, direction and friendship.

My writing life has been enriched by the Saltwater Writers'

Circle. Thank you for inspiration and critical listening to Jesse Bown (tens of thousands of kilometres of conversation and joy), Dorothy Harvey (the Freshwater poet and muse), Pat Collins (Harbour Grace's foremost historian) and Angie Green (who always understands).

I am grateful for the early encouragement from the wonderful Newfoundland writer Jessica Grant. Small kindnesses can have surprisingly profound repercussions. I can only hope to show the same helpfulness to others.

My agent, Robert Mackwood of Seventh Avenue Literary Agency, believed in *Creatures*. Without his interest and work this book would not be.

Editor Tim Rostron of Doubleday Canada understood these stories from the start. His skill, wit and care have been a big part of *Creatures of the Rock*. Thank you, Tim, for your direction and thoughtful work on the book. Thanks also to line editor Shaun Oakey for his meticulous attention to detail.

My parents, Jackson and Susan Peacock, encouraged my brothers and me to read and think about what we read from when we were very small. Our home was always a place of books; perhaps it was inevitable that a couple of writers emerged. Thanks for everything, Dad, Shane, Mark and Stephen. I know Mom would have been proud to see this book.

Liam, Adrian and Astrid, of course you are stars of the book. Thanks for helping make the story and for your reading and support during my writing.

My biggest thanks goes to my best friend. Ingrid was, is and will always be a big part of all of my stories. She's the first reader of everything I write and always full of helpful ideas and encouragement. As we would say in Newfoundland—I certainly could have done a lot worse.